NUTRITION
A KEY TO GOOD HEALTH

NUTRITION
A KEY TO GOOD HEALTH

Susan Narayan

INFORMATION PLUS® REFERENCE SERIES
Formerly published by Information Plus, Wylie, Texas

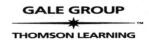

GALE GROUP
THOMSON LEARNING

Detroit • New York • San Diego • San Francisco
Boston • New Haven, Conn. • Waterville, Maine
London • Munich

NUTRITION: A KEY TO GOOD HEALTH

Susan Narayan, *Author*

The Gale Group Staff:

Editorial: Ellice Engdahl, *Series Editor*; John F. McCoy, *Series Editor*; Charles B. Montney, *Series Editor*; Andrew Claps, *Series Associate Editor*; Jason M. Everett, *Series Associate Editor*; Michael T. Reade, *Series Associate Editor*; Heather Price, *Series Assistant Editor*; Teresa Elsey, *Editorial Assistant*; Debra M. Kirby, *Managing Editor*; Rita Runchock, *Managing Editor*

Image and Multimedia Content: Barbara J. Yarrow, *Manager, Imaging and Multimedia Content*; Robyn Young, *Project Manager, Imaging and Multimedia Content*

Indexing: Amy Suchowski, *Indexing Specialist*

Permissions: Margaret Chamberlain, *Permissions Specialist*; Maria Franklin, *Permissions Manager*

Product Design: Michelle DiMercurio, *Senior Art Director and Product Design Manager*; Michael Logusz, *Cover Art Designer*

Production: Evi Seoud, *Assistant Manager, Composition Purchasing and Electronic Prepress*; NeKita McKee, *Buyer*; Dorothy Maki, *Manufacturing Manager*

Cover photo © PhotoDisk

ISBN 0-7876-5103-6 (set)
ISBN 0-7876-5401-9 (this volume)
ISSN 1536-5255 (this volume)
Printed in the United States of America
10 9 8 7 6 5 4 3 2 1

TABLE OF CONTENTS

America's nutrients come from the products of its farms; yet, the number of farms and farmers decreases every year. This chapter draws a statistical picture of the American farm and discusses recent trends in agriculture.

The American diet has varied over time. This chapter reports on what and how much Americans eat, and explains the reasons for recent changes.

People are becoming more conscious of the effects various foods can have on their health, and often are altering their consumption patterns to reflect this. The government provides guidelines to help Americans make appropriate dietary choices. This chapter outlines these guidelines and discusses significant issues related to nutrient intake.

Before food can be consumed, it must be purchased. This chapter explores how much people pay for food, whether the poor pay more, and how the American food dollar is spent.

Many people do their food shopping at supermarkets. This chapter provides statistics on average grocery spending, the attitude of consumers toward prepared food and other services offered by supermarkets, and the influence of nutrition considerations on food purchasing decisions.

Mandatory food labeling allows consumers to make informed choices about the nutrient content of the foods they purchase. This chapter outlines government requirements for nutrition labeling and other label claims.

Foodborne pathogens have always been a safety concern. New food technologies and innovations, including biotechnology, novel macro-ingredients, functional foods, and irradiation, create new questions about food safety. Pesticide residue monitoring, organic foods, and dietary supplements are also discussed in this chapter.

More people than ever are aware of the health benefits of a nutritious diet, but many have not significantly improved their eating habits. Studies show that people's perceptions of what they eat differ from what they actually eat and that their knowledge about nutrition may be incomplete. This chapter also explores shopper attitudes toward self-care and the impact of eating out on nutrition.

Increasing numbers of Americans are overweight or obese. This chapter outlines the causes and consequences of obesity and examines dieting. Diet drugs, eating disorders, and exercise are also discussed.

Though most Americans are sufficiently well-fed, some still suffer from hunger or food insecurity. This chapter describes the federal programs dedicated to providing adequate nutrition to all.

PREFACE

Nutrition: A Key to Good Health is one of the latest volumes in the Information Plus Reference Series. Previously published by the Information Plus company of Wylie, Texas, the Information Plus Reference Series (and its companion set, the Information Plus Compact Series) became a Gale Group product when Gale and Information Plus merged in early 2000. Those of you familiar with the series as published by Information Plus will notice a few changes from the 1999 edition. Gale has adopted a new layout and style that we hope you will find easy to use. Other improvements include greatly expanded indexes in each book, and more descriptive tables of contents.

While some changes have been made to the design, the purpose of the Information Plus Reference Series remains the same. Each volume of the series presents the latest facts on a topic of pressing concern in modern American life. These topics include today's most controversial and most studied social issues: abortion, capital punishment, care for the elderly, crime, health care, the environment, immigration, minorities, social welfare, women, youth, and many more. Although written especially for the high school and undergraduate student, this series is an excellent resource for anyone in need of factual information on current affairs.

By presenting the facts, it is Gale's intention to provide its readers with everything they need to reach an informed opinion on current issues. To that end, there is a particular emphasis in this series on the presentation of scientific studies, surveys, and statistics. These data are generally presented in the form of tables, charts, and other graphics placed within the text of each book. Every graphic is directly referred to and carefully explained in the text. The source of each graphic is presented within the graphic itself. The data used in these graphics is drawn from the most reputable and reliable sources, in particular the various branches of the U.S. government and major independent polling organizations. Every effort has been made to secure the most recent information available. The reader should bear in mind that many major studies take years to conduct, and that additional years often pass before the data from these studies is made available to the public. Therefore, in many cases the most recent information available in 2001 is dated from 1998 or 1999. Older statistics are sometimes presented as well, if they are of particular interest and no more recent information exists.

Although statistics are a major focus of the Information Plus Reference Series, they are by no means its only content. Each book also presents the widely held positions and important ideas that shape how the book's subject is discussed in the United States. These positions are explained in detail and, where possible, in the words of their proponents. Some of the other material to be found in these books includes: historical background; descriptions of major events related to the subject; relevant laws and court cases; and examples of how these issues play out in American life. Some books also feature primary documents, or have pro and con debate sections giving the words and opinions of prominent Americans on both sides of a controversial topic. All material is presented in an even-handed and unbiased manner; the reader will never be encouraged to accept one view of an issue over another.

HOW TO USE THIS BOOK

Food and nutrition are subjects of vital importance to everyone. Nutritionists, doctors, and psychologists are constantly studying the effects of diet on a person's body and mind, while economists and businessmen study the food purchasing habits of consumers. As result of this research, our understanding of what Americans should eat, what they actually eat, and why, is constantly changing. This book presents the most recent research on major nutrition and nutrition-related topics, with a particular emphasis on controversial or rapidly changing areas, such as obesity among Americans, food safety, eating disorders, and the ever-changing definition of a healthy diet.

Nutrition: A Key to Good Health consists of ten chapters and three appendices. Each chapter is devoted to a particular nutrition or food related issue. For a summary of the information covered in each chapter, please see the synopses provided in the Table of Contents at the front of the book. Chapters generally begin with an overview of the basic facts and background information on the chapter's topic, then proceed to examine sub-topics of particular interest. For example, Chapter 6: Food Labeling begins with a history of government involvement in food labeling and health claims, explaining how the current regulatory system came about. It then describes the government's nutrition label, what it is for, and what its various parts mean. From there, the chapter moves on to describe how the government regulates health claims on food packaging, as well as other common claims such as "light," or "healthy." Then the chapter describes exceptions to the normal labeling rules, and concludes with statistics on whether or not people actually pay attention to nutritional labeling. Readers can find their way through a chapter by looking for the section and sub-section headings, which are clearly set off from the text. Or, they can refer to the book's extensive index if they already know what they are looking for.

Statistical Information

The tables and figures featured throughout *Nutrition: A Key to Good Health* will be of particular use to the reader in learning about this issue. These tables and figures represent an extensive collection of the most recent, interesting, and important statistics on nutrition and related issues—for example, the amount of fat in a typical American's diet, the recommended calorie intake for men and women of different ages and activity levels, the percentage of Americans who say they would avoid purchasing bioengineered foods, and the number of Americans who receive government food assistance. Gale believes that making this information available to the reader is the most

important way in which we fulfill the goal of this book: to help readers understand the issues and controversies surrounding food and nutrition in the United States and reach their own conclusions.

Each table or figure has a unique identifier appearing above it, for ease of identification and reference. Titles for the tables and figures explain their purpose. At the end of each table or figure, the original source of the data is provided.

In order to help readers understand these often complicated statistics, all tables and figures are explained in the text. References in the text direct the reader to the relevant statistics. Furthermore, the contents of all tables and figures are fully indexed. Please see the opening section of the index at the back of this volume for a description of how to find tables and figures within it.

In addition to the main body text and images, *Nutrition: A Key to Good Health* has three appendices. The first is the Important Names and Addresses directory. Here the reader will find contact information for a number of government and private organizations that can provide information on food and nutrition. The second appendix is the Resources section, which can also assist the reader in conducting his or her own research. In this section, the author and editors of *Nutrition: A Key to Good Health* describe some of the sources that were most useful during the compilation of this book. The final appendix is the index. It has been greatly expanded from previous editions, and should make it even easier to find specific topics in this book.

COMMENTS AND SUGGESTIONS

The editors of the Information Plus Reference Series welcome your feedback on *Nutrition: A Key to Good Health*. Please direct all correspondence to:

Editor
Information Plus Reference Series
27500 Drake Rd.
Farmington Hills, MI, 48331-3535

ACKNOWLEDGEMENTS

Following is a list of the copyright holders who have granted us permission to reproduce material in Information Plus: Nutrition. *Every effort has been made to trace copyright, but if omissions have been made, please let us know.*

Food Marketing Institute, and PREVENTION Magazine. *A Shopping for Health Report, 1998: A Look at the Self-Care Movement.* Reproduced by permission.

Food Marketing Institute and PREVENTION Magazine. "Attitudes Toward Prepared Food," in *A Shopping for Health Report, 1998: Consumer Interest in Nutritious Prepared.* Reproduced by permission.

National Academy of Sciences, Washington DC. "Recommended Levels for Individual Intake, 1998, B Vitamins and Choline." Reproduced by permission of National Academy Press.

Wheat Foods Council, Parker, CO. *Setting the Record Straight: What America Thinks About Fad Diets, Nutrition Advice and Food.* Reproduced by permission.

Centers for Disease Control. Illustration from: *Food-Related Illness and Death in the U.S.,* (1999)

Centers for Disease Control. Illustrations from: *Morbidity and Mortality Weekly Report* April 21, 2000; March 9, 2001

Centers for Disease Control and Prevention, National Center for Health Studies. Illustrations from: *Prevalence of Overweight Among Children and Adolescents: United States, 1999* and *Prevalence of Overweight and Obesity Among Adults: United States, 1999*

Environmental Working Group Illustrations from: *How 'Bout Them Apples? Pesticides in Children's Food Ten Years After,* (1999)

Food Marketing Institute. Illustrations from: *Trends in the United States: Consumer Attitudes & the Supermarket 2000,* (2000)

National Academy of Sciences, Food Nutrition Board. Illlustrations from: "Dietary Reference Intakes (RDI)" (1998) and "Recommended Energy Intake" in "Recommended Daily Allowances"

National Agricultural Statistics Service. Illustration from: "Distribution of Farms and Land in Farms, by Region, 1999" (2000)

National Institutes of Health, Office of Dietary Supplements, Clinical Nutrition Service. Illustration from: *Facts About Dietary Supplements,* (2000)

National Institutes of Health, National Heart, Lung, and Blood Institute. Illustrations from: *Clinical Guidelines on the Identification, Evaluation, and Treatment of Overweight and Obesity in Adults, 1998*

National Institutes of Health, National Heart, Lung, and Blood Institute, National High Blood Pressure Education Program. Illustrations from: *Facts About Lowering Blood Pressure,* (2000)

National Institutes of Health, Weight Control Information Network. Illustration from: *Statistics Related to Overweight and Obesity,* (2000)

Oklahoma State University, Division of Agricultural Sciences and Natural Resources, Oklahoma Cooperative Extension Service. Illustration from: *Dietary Fiber,* May 1999

U.S. Census Bureau. Illustration from: *Statistical Abstract of the United States, 2000,* (2000)

U.S. Department of Agriculture. Illustrations from: *Agricultural Fact Book 2000* (2000) *Dietary Guidelines for Americans, 2000* (2000), *Food Consumption, Prices and Expenditures, 1970–1997* (1998), *The Food Guide Pyramid for Young Children* (1999), and *Nutrition and Your Health: Dietary Guidelines for Americans,* (2000)

U.S. Department of Agriculture, Center for Nutrition Policy and Promotion. Illustrations from: *Food Guide Pyramid Booklet 2000* (2000), *Nutrition Insights,* (1997), *Beliefs and Attitudes of Americans Toward their Diet,* Nutrition Insights 19, (2000), and *Consumption of Food Group Servings: People's Perceptions vs. Reality,* (2000) Nutrition Insights 20

U.S. Department of Agriculture, Center for Nutrition Policy and Promotion. Illustration from: *Report Card on the Diet Quality of African Americans,* (1998)

U.S. Department of Agriculture, Economic Research Service. Illustrations from: *FoodReview* Vol. 21, Issue 3, August 1999; Vol. 22, Issue 3, Sept-Dec., 1999; Volume 23, Issue 3, March 2001

U.S. Department of Agriculture, Economic Research Service. Illustrations from: *Agricultural Outlook,* April 2000, and *USDA Agricultural Projections to 2010,* February 2001

U.S. Department of Agriculture, Economic Research Service. Illustration from: *USDA's Healthy Eating Index and Nutrition Information,* (1998) Technical Bulletin No. 1866

U.S. Department of Agriculture, Economic Research Service. Illustrations from: *A Comparison of Food Assistance Programs in Mexico and the U.S.* and *Household Food Security in the U.S., 1999* (2000), Food Assistance and Nutrition Research Report No. 6

U.S. Department of Agriculture, Food and Nutrition Service. Illustration from: *WIC Participation and Program Characteristics 1998,* May 2000

U.S. Department of Agriculture, Food and Drug Administration, Economic Research Service. Illustration from: *Away-From-Home-Foods Increasingly Important to Quality of American Diet,* Agricultural Information Bulletin # 749, 2000

U.S. Food and Drug Administration. Illustrations from: *Food Labeling Guide,* June 1999,

An FDA Guide to Dietary Supplements, 1999, and *FDA Consumer,* Jan.-Feb., 1999

U.S. Food and Drug Administration, FDA Pesticide Program: Residue Monitoring, 1999

U.S. Food and Drug Administration, Center for Food Safety and Applied Nutrition. Illustrations from: *Foodborne Pathogenic*

Microorganisms and Natural Toxins Handbook, 1999, and *Guidance on How to Understand and Use the Nutrition Facts Panel on Food Labels,* June 2000

U.S. General Accounting Office. Illustrations from: *Food Irradiation: Available Research Indicates that Benefits Outweigh Risks,* (2000)

CHAPTER 1
AGRICULTURE

The farm has long held a cherished place in American tradition. The wholesome, hard-working family raising corn or cattle has often been mythically portrayed as the backbone of the "heartland of America." Americans have frequently looked upon the farmer and rancher as the creators of this country's bounty. Today, farming is undergoing a major transformation as fewer, larger farms produce food with the help of high-technology mechanization, not family members.

THE *1997 CENSUS OF AGRICULTURE*

The Bureau of the Census of the U.S. Department of Commerce conducted the first agriculture census in 1840 as part of the fifth decennial (occurring every ten years) population census. Other agriculture censuses were taken as Congress saw fit. Beginning in 1982 the agricultural census has been taken every five years. For the first time, in 1997, the Bureau of the Census turned over the responsibility of conducting the *1997 Census of Agriculture* (National Agricultural Statistics Service, U.S. Department of Agriculture, Washington, D.C., 1999) to the National Agricultural Statistics Service (NASS) of the U.S. Department of Agriculture (USDA).

PORTRAIT OF FARMS

The *1997 Census of Agriculture* counted 1,911,859 farms in the United States, slightly less than in 1992. For the purpose of the census, a farm is "any place from which $1,000 or more of agricultural products were produced and sold, or normally would have been produced and sold, during the census year." The average farm size increased from 462 acres in 1987 to 487 acres in 1997. The amount of land in farms (farmlands) continued to decline, down to about 932 million acres in 1997, from about 964 million acres in 1987 (See Table 1.1) and from its peak of 1.2 billion acres in 1954 (not shown). Figure 1.1 shows the land in farms by state.

FIGURE 1.1

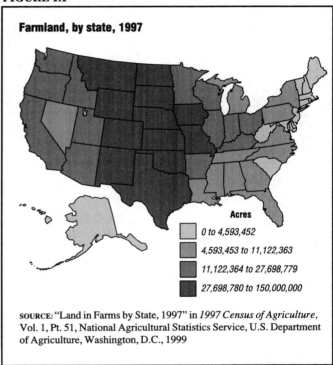

Farmland, by state, 1997

Acres
- 0 to 4,593,452
- 4,593,453 to 11,122,363
- 11,122,364 to 27,698,779
- 27,698,780 to 150,000,000

SOURCE: "Land in Farms by State, 1997" in *1997 Census of Agriculture,* Vol. 1, Pt. 51, National Agricultural Statistics Service, U.S. Department of Agriculture, Washington, D.C., 1999

Of the 932 million acres of farmlands in 1997, 46.3 percent accounted for cropland and 42.5 percent for pastureland and rangeland. Of the 431 million acres of cropland, 71.8 percent was used for harvested crops, and 8.8 percent was used for cover crops, had failed crops, or was summer-fallowed (plowed and tilled but left unseeded). About 4.4 percent remained idle, and 15 percent was used for pasture. (See Figure 1.2.)

In 1997 many (60.5 percent) farms were small—between 1 and 179 acres in size. (See Figure 1.3.) Half (50.3 percent) of all farms, however, sold less than $10,000 and accounted for only 1.5 percent of total farm sales. Conversely, farms with sales of $500,000 or more made up

TABLE 1.1

Census of Agriculture historical highlights: 1964–97

All items		1997	1992	1987	1982	1978	1974	1969	1964
Farms number		1,911,859	1,925,300	2,087,759	2,240,976	2,257,775	2,314,013	2,730,250	3,157,857
Land in farms	acres	931,795,255	945,531,506	964,470,625	986,796,579	1,014,777,234	1,017,030,357	1,062,892,501	1,110,187,000
Average size of farm	acres	487	491	462	440	449	440	389	352
Estimated market value of land and buildings[1]									
Average per farm	dollars	449,748	357,056	289,387	345,869	279,672	147,838	75,714	50,646
Average per acre	dollars	933	727	627	784	619	336	194	144
Estimated market value of all machinery and equipment[1]	$1,000	110,256,802	93,316,496	85,801,360	93,662,947	77,600,689	48,402,624	25, 343,077	(NA)
Average per farm	dollars	57,678	48,605	41,227	41,919	34,471	22,303	9,770	(NA)
Farms by size									
1 to 9 acres		153,515	166,496	183,257	187,665	151,233	128,254	162,111	182,581
10 to 49 acres		410,833	387,711	412,437	449,252	391,554	379,543	473,465	637,434
50 to 179 acres		592,972	584,146	644,849	711,652	759,047	827,884	1,001,706	1,175,370
180 to 499 acres		402,769	427,648	478,294	526,510	581,631	616,098	726,363	806,743
500 to 999 acres		175,690	186,387	200,058	203,925	213,209	207,297	215,659	210,437
1,000 to 1,999 acres		101,468	101,923	102,078	97,395	97,800	92,712	91,039	84,999
2,000 acres or more		74,612	70,989	66,786	64,577	63,301	62,225	59,907	60,293
Total cropland	farms	1,661,395	1,697,137	1,848,574	2,010,609	2,081,604	2,157,511	2,521,659	2,907,265
	acres	431,144,896	435,365,878	443,318,233	445,362,028	453,874,133	440,039,087	458,989,605	434,232,200
Harvested cropland	farms	1,410,606	1,491,786	1,643,633	1,809,756	1,904,602	1,954,700	2,219,631	2,701,694
	acres	309,395,475	295,936,976	282,223,880	326,306,462	317,145,955	303,001,943	273,016,000	286,891,974
Irrigated land	farms	279,442	279,357	291,628	278,277	280,779	236,733	257,147	297,387
	acres	55,058,128	49,404,030	46,386,201	49,002,433	50,349,906	41,243,023	39,121,693	37,056,083
Market value of agricultural products sold[2]	$1,000	196,864,649	162,608,334	136,048,516	131,900,223	107,073,458	81,526,126	45,563,891	35,292,431
Average per farm	dollars	102,970	84,459	65,165	58,858	47,424	35,231	16,689	11,176
Crops, including nursery and greenhouse crops	$1,000	98,055,656	75,228,256	58,931,085	62,256,087	48,203,200	41,790,365	16,922,023	16,236,248
Livestock, poultry, and their products	$1,000	98,808,993	87,380,078	77,117,431	69,644,136	58,870,258	39,503,850	28,480,921	18,841,027
Farms by value of sales[3]									
Less than $2,500		496,514	422,767	490,296	536,327	460,535	649,448	1,031,638	1,338,259
$2,500 to $4,999		228,477	231,867	262,918	278,208	300,699	257,263	357,922	443,918
$5,000 to $9,999		237,975	251,883	274,972	281,802	314,088	296,373	390,425	504,614
$10,000 to $24,999		274,040	301,804	326,166	340,254	394,876	956,092	896,159	837,507
$25,000 to $49,999		170,705	195,354	219,636	248,828	300,515			
$50,000 to $99,999		158,160	187,760	218,050	251,501	263,092			
$100,000 to $499,999		277,194	286,951	263,698	274,580	203,695	141,187	47,916	31,401
$500,000 or more		68,794	46,914	32,023	27,800	17,973	11,412	4,079	
Farms by type of organization									
Individual or family (sole proprietorship)		1,643,424	1,653,491	1,809,324	1,945,639	1,965,860	(NA)	(NA)	(NA)
Partnership		169,462	186,806	199,559	223,274	232,538	(NA)	(NA)	(NA)
Corporation		84,002	72,567	66,969	59,792	50,231	(NA)	(NA)	(NA)
Other—cooperative, estate or trust, institutional, etc.		14,971	12,436	11,907	12,271	9,146	(NA)	(NA)	(NA)
Operators by days worked off farm[4]									
None		755,254	801,881	844,476	861,798	942,803	829,843	(NA)	(NA)
Any		1,042,158	992,773	1,115,560	1,187,374	1,203,286	1,011,476	1,482,292	1,462,183
200 days or more		709,279	665,570	737,206	774,844	770,045	657,971	870,815	824,173
Operators by principal occupation[4]									
Farming		961,560	1,053,150	1,138,179	1,234,787	1,269,305	1,427,368	(NA)	(NA)
Other		950,299	872,150	949,580	1,006,189	988,470	851,902	(NA)	(NA)
Average age of operator[4]	years	54.3	53.3	52.0	50.5	50.3	51.7	51.2	51.3
Total farm production expenses[1]	$1,000	150,590,993	130,779,261	108,138,053	(NA)	(NA)	61,007,649	37,559,615	(NA)
Selected farm production expenses[1]									
Livestock and poultry purchased	$1,000	21,614,559	23,043.431	19,344,645	17,174,334	16,039,244	9,953,946	8,077,779	4,177,785
Feed for livestock and poultry	$1,000	32,759,966	24,084,507	19,163,364	18,591,984	15,785,995	13,647,816	7,082,274	5,511,813

TABLE 1.1

Census of Agriculture historical highlights: 1964–97 [CONTINUED]

All items		1997	1992	1987	1982	1978	1974	1969	1964
Selected farm production (continued)									
Commercial fertilizer[5]	$1,000	9,597,128	8,204,324	6,684,944	7,689,365	6,330,581	5,137,361	2,209,185	1,771,617
Petroleum products	$1,000	6,371,515	6,120,452	5,277,227	7,888,052	4,691,425	3,087,606	1,906,579	1,786,796
Hired farm labor	$1,000	14,841,036	12,961,639	10,866,236	8,441,180	6,814,428	4,652,075	3,375,203	2,798,571
Interest[6]	$1,000	8,928,107	8,111,337	8,158,268	11,668,942	(NA)	(NA)	(NA)	(NA)
Agricultural chemicals[5]	$1,000	7,581,424	6,133,705	4,690,243	4,282,213	2,889,503	1,757,779	908,036	(NA)
Livestock and poultry									
Cattle and calves									
inventory	farms	1,046,863	1,074,349	1,176,346	1,354,992	1,346,106	1,503,244	1,719,403	2,283,881
	number	98,989,244	96,135,825	95,847,299	104,475,827	103,865,109	113,174,700	106,345,741	105,557,830
Beef cows	farms	804,595	803,241	841,778	957,698	954,360	1,024,935		1,323,912
	number	34,066,615	32,545,976	31,652,593	34,202,607	34,326,274	41,257,898	34,337,320	32,719,198
Milk cows	farms	116,874	155,339	202,068	277,762	312,095	403,754	568,237	1,133,912
	number	9,095,439	9,491,818	10,084,697	10,849,890	10,221,692	10,654,516	11,174,036	14,622,604
Cattle and calves sold	farms	1,011,809	1,034,189	1,150,523	1,278,609	1,320,163	1,437,101	1,645,518	1,990,968
	number	74,089,046	70,562,908	72,603,841	71,216,727	78,020,351	70,019,180	74,616,155	62,952,104
Hogs and pigs inventory	farms	109,754	191,347	243,398	329,833	445,117	470,258	686,097	1,081,438
	number	61,206,236	57,563,118	52,271,120	55,366,205	57,697,318	45,503,604	55,454,828	54,080,194
Hogs and pigs sold	farms	102,106	188,167	238,819	315,095	423,578	449,841	645,129	802,620
	number	142,611,882	111,326,807	96,569,359	94,783,598	90,757,143	79,897,397	89,313,449	83,537,060
Layers and pullets 13 weeks old and older inventory (see text)[7]	farms	72,616	88,235	144,438	215,812	240,891	316,243	471,284	1,210,669
	number	366,989,851	351,310,317	373,577,186	362,464,997	354,357,427	335,740,245	371,008,459	343,161,807
Broilers and other meat-type chickens sold	farms	23,937	23,949	27,645	30,100	31,743	34,340	33,753	35,128
	number	6,741,927,110	5,428,589,485	4,361,975,630	3,516,622,889	3,062,154,490	2,518,513,032	2,429,773,426	1,915,373,928
Selected crops harvested									
Corn for grain or seed	farms	430,711	503,935	627,602	715,171	810,577	883,309	985,629	1,382,773
	acres	69,796,716	69,339,869	58,701,505	69,857,993	70,043,480	61,653,842	52,540,249	53,751,095
	bushels	8,578,634,770	8,697,362,804	6,725,001,837	7,508,721,493	6,805,185,861	4,396,912,922	4,441,808,244	3,361,141,669
Wheat for grain	farms	243,568	292,464	352,237	446,075	378,574	533,520	583,605	739,662
	acres	58,836,344	59,089,470	53,224,174	70,910,293	54,155,168	62,957,215	45,372,868	47,958,362
	bushels	2,204,026,684	2,206,729,476	1,887,103,964	2,373,246,659	1,607,540,430	1,691,553,354	1,328,003,477	1,217,791,875
Soybeans for beans	farms	354,692	381,000	441,899	511,229	537,037	542,029	529,798	560,156
	acres	66,147,726	56,351,304	55,291,205	64,832,842	61,339,849	48,118,849	38,549,663	29,843,540
	bushels	2,504,307,294	2,053,163,265	1,838,053,979	1,989,993,158	1,722,154,229	1,145,788,470	1,041,489,049	669,664,562
Cotton	farms	31,493	34,812	43,046	38,266	52,628	89,536	199,785	324,361
	acres	13,235,236	10,961,720	9,826,081	9,781,404	12,693,772	12,223,500	11,496,220	13,916,648
	bales	17,878,743	15,370,310	13,280,143	11,375,524	10,,686,447	10,887,205	10,360,171	14,734,217
Tobacco	farms	89,706	124,270	136,682	179,141	188,649	197,764	276,188	331,365
	acres	838,530	831,231	633,310	931,655	963,224	877,113	876,927	1,025,240
	pounds	1,747,702,321	1,697,831,562	1,215,221,360	1,871,309,459	1,918,189,782	1,733,365,121	1,643,934,800	1,987,526,982
Hay –alfalfa, other tame, small grain, wild, grass silage, green chop, etc. (see text)	farms	888,597	905,296	994,551	1,050,992	1,132,997	1,145,540	1,229,877	(NA)
	acres	60,799,788	56,596,466	57,967,530	56,743,836	60,241,391	56,236,381	53,203,606	65,294,703
	tons, dry	139,365,313	126,981,302	128,816,054	128,474,661	130,713,685	115,028,236	111,813,581	115,760,894
Vegetables harvested for sale (see text)[8]	farms	53,727	61,969	60,819	69,109	73,183	78,566	101,760	131,653
	acres	3,773,219	3,782,358	3,467,563	3,330,637	3,534,142	3,124,257	3,352,385	3,333,772
Land in orchards	farms	106,069	116,207	120,434	123,663	121,852	105,997	133,311	224,568
	acres	5,158,064	4,770,778	4,560,183	4,750,667	4,463,627	4,190,340	4,233,897	4,251,130

[1]Data are based on a sample of farms.
[2]Data for 1974 and prior years include the value of forest products sold.
[3]Data for 1982 and prior years exclude abnormal farms
[4]Data for 1974 apply only to individual or family operations (sole proprietorship) and partnerships.
[5]Data for 1964 to 1982 do not include cost of custom applications; data for agricultural chemicals include the cost of lime for 1969 to 1978.
[6]Data for 1982 do not include imputation for item nonresponse.
[7]Data for 1969 to 1992 are for chickens 3 months old or older inventory; data for 1964 are for chickens 4 months old or older .
[8]Data for 1974 were from land area used.

SOURCE: "Historical Highlights: 1997 and Earlier Census Years" in *1997 Census of Agriculture*, Vol. 1, Pt. 51, National Agricultural Statistics Service, U.S. Department of Agriculture, Washington, D.C., 1999

FIGURE 1.2

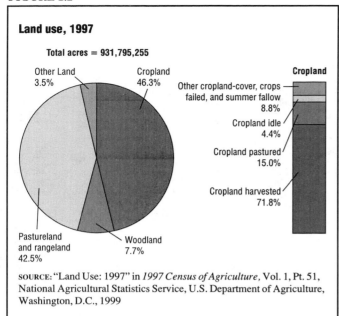

Land use, 1997

Total acres = 931,795,255

SOURCE: "Land Use: 1997" in *1997 Census of Agriculture,* Vol. 1, Pt. 51, National Agricultural Statistics Service, U.S. Department of Agriculture, Washington, D.C., 1999

only 3.6 percent of all farms but accounted for more than half (56.6 percent) of all sales. (See Figure 1.4.) The total market value of agricultural products (crops as well as livestock, poultry, and their products) sold in 1997 reached $196.9 billion, up 45 percent since 1987 ($136 billion). The average sales per farm were $102,970, up 58 percent from $65,165 in 1987. (See Table 1.1.)

Farm Numbers in 1999

In addition to conducting the *1997 Census of Agriculture,* the NASS continues to administer the collection and publication of timely national and state agricultural statistics. The NASS reports that in 1999 there were 2.19 million farms in the United States, up from 2.14 million in 1990. The average farm size decreased from 460 to 432 acres during that time period. Land in farms also decreased—from 986 million acres in 1990 to 947 million acres in 1999. Figure 1.5 shows the distribution of farms and land in farms in the different regions of the country. For example, the South had 42 percent of farms in the United States and 30 percent of farmlands.

WHO GROWS AMERICA'S FOOD?

Fewer Farmers

Until the Industrial Revolution, the U.S. economy was mainly agricultural. In 1810, 84 percent of the labor force worked in farming. By 1950, 12.2 percent of the labor force worked in farming. In 2000 farmers accounted for only 2.4 percent of the workforce. The mass exodus from farming occurred mostly in the 1970s.

In 1998 family workers, including farm operators and unpaid workers, made up 69 percent of farm labor. Hired

farm workers accounted for the remaining 31 percent. Service workers, including crew leaders and custom crews (workers who provided skilled labor and their own equipment), made up 9 percent of all workers on farms.

Several key factors have driven workers out of farming. Technological advances, such as the increased use of fertilization, improved irrigation, and larger tractor equipment, have led to dramatic increases in productivity and reductions in employment. Relatively high costs of land and equipment have restricted access to farming for many and forced others to abandon farming. The expansion of the service sector created a demand for labor in nonfarm industries, and higher earnings attracted many workers away from agriculture. On the other hand, Hispanic immigration, largely from Mexico, has provided a large pool of low-wage agricultural labor.

Since the 1970s dramatic changes have been seen in farming—from the use of black farm workers to Hispanic workers, from smaller to larger farms, from lower to higher levels of educational attainment, and, to some extent, from male to female ownership. Finally, unpaid work by family members, which was once typical in farms, has declined substantially.

WHAT AMERICA GROWS

Crops

America's beautiful "amber waves of grain" are most likely to be cornfields and soybean fields. Corn is not only the largest crop produced, but it is also the nation's largest export. Farmers harvested 70.5 million acres of corn, 72.4 million acres of soybeans, and 53.8 million acres of wheat in 1999. Another 26.3 million acres harvested were of cotton, sorghum, and barley.

Livestock and Poultry

In 1997 livestock and poultry sales in the United States totaled $98.8 billion. Nearly half the livestock value was in cattle and calves (41 percent). Poultry and poultry products made up 22.5 percent; dairy products, 19.2 percent; and hogs and pigs, 14 percent. (See Figure 1.6.)

As people's incomes rise, they usually demand a higher-quality diet that often includes animal products. Years ago chickens were raised mainly for egg production. The meat from chickens was only a by-product of egg production. Chickens were often scavengers, eating feed and other things that could be found around the farmyard, such as insects. Because chickens were used mainly for egg laying, chicken meat was expensive, compared to the price of pork and beef.

Then growers changed the way chickens were raised, putting them in environmentally controlled conditions. This was called confinement production. The growers kept the newly developed hybrid chickens in small areas

FIGURE 1.3

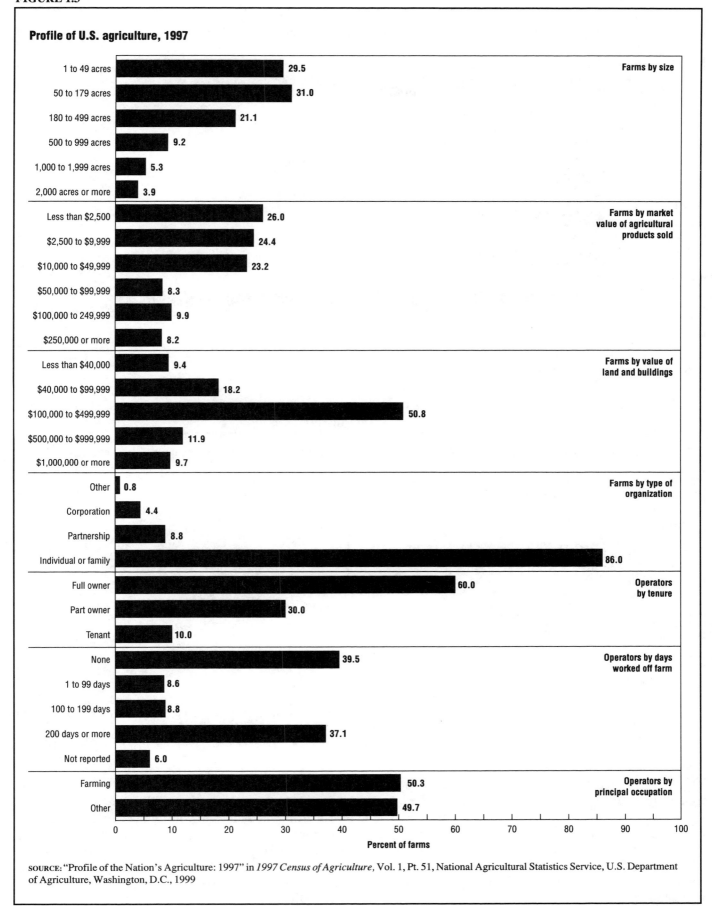

Profile of U.S. agriculture, 1997

SOURCE: "Profile of the Nation's Agriculture: 1997" in *1997 Census of Agriculture,* Vol. 1, Pt. 51, National Agricultural Statistics Service, U.S. Department of Agriculture, Washington, D.C., 1999

FIGURE 1.4

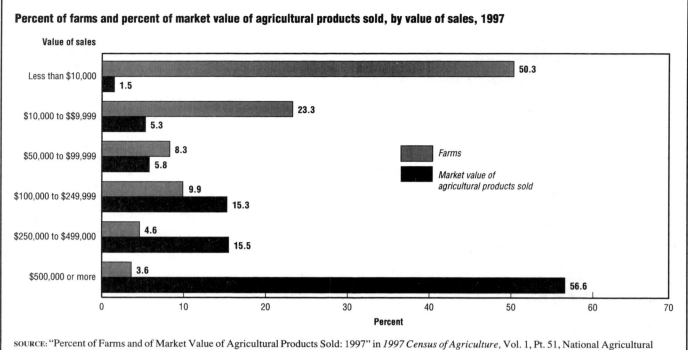

Percent of farms and percent of market value of agricultural products sold, by value of sales, 1997

Value of sales

Less than $10,000	Farms: 50.3	Market value: 1.5
$10,000 to $$9,999	Farms: 23.3	Market value: 5.3
$50,000 to $99,999	Farms: 8.3	Market value: 5.8
$100,000 to $249,999	Farms: 9.9	Market value: 15.3
$250,000 to $499,000	Farms: 4.6	Market value: 15.5
$500,000 or more	Farms: 3.6	Market value: 56.6

■ Farms
■ Market value of agricultural products sold

Percent (0, 10, 20, 30, 40, 50, 60, 70)

SOURCE: "Percent of Farms and of Market Value of Agricultural Products Sold: 1997" in *1997 Census of Agriculture,* Vol. 1, Pt. 51, National Agricultural Statistics Service, U.S. Department of Agriculture, Washington, D.C., 1999

FIGURE 1.5

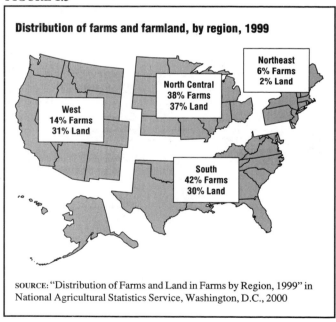

Distribution of farms and farmland, by region, 1999

Northeast
6% Farms
2% Land

North Central
38% Farms
37% Land

West
14% Farms
31% Land

South
42% Farms
30% Land

SOURCE: "Distribution of Farms and Land in Farms by Region, 1999" in National Agricultural Statistics Service, Washington, D.C., 2000

FIGURE 1.6

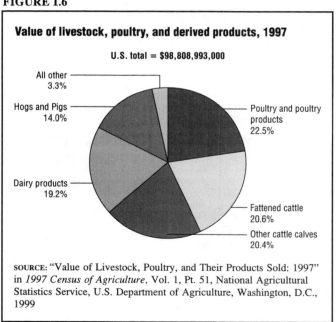

Value of livestock, poultry, and derived products, 1997

U.S. total = $98,808,993,000

All other
3.3%

Hogs and Pigs
14.0%

Dairy products
19.2%

Poultry and poultry products
22.5%

Fattened cattle
20.6%

Other cattle calves
20.4%

SOURCE: "Value of Livestock, Poultry, and Their Products Sold: 1997" in *1997 Census of Agriculture,* Vol. 1, Pt. 51, National Agricultural Statistics Service, U.S. Department of Agriculture, Washington, D.C., 1999

and fed them high-quality grains. Drugs reduced losses from disease, making confinement possible. This resulted in lower prices for chicken meat so that more people could afford it. Close control of all production stages, from feed preparation to slaughter, further reduced costs. Chicken has become one of the least expensive meats a person can buy, with the price declining by about two-thirds from the mid-1950s.

Raising swine (hogs) for pork production has also changed. As with chickens, confining the hogs in small areas, using medicines to control disease, feeding them better food, and managing farms more efficiently have increased pork production not just in the United States but around the world. In fact, more pork is sold on the world market than beef, while chicken is gaining in popularity.

TABLE 1.2

Growth in organic agriculture, 1992–97

U.S. certified organic	1992	1993	1994	1995	1996	1997	Change 1992-97	1995-97
				1,000 acres			Percent	
Farmland								
Total	935	956	992	918	—	1,347	44	47
Pasture & rangeland	532	491	435	279	—	496	-7	78
Cropland	403	465	557	639	—	850	111	33
				Number			Percent	
Animals								
Beef cows	6,796	9,222	3,300	—	—	4,429	-35	—
Milk cows	2,265	2,846	6,100	—	—	12,897	469	—
Hogs and pigs	1,365	1,499	2,100	—	—	482	-65	—
Sheep and lambs	1,221	1,186	1,600	—	—	705	-42	—
Layer hens	43,981	20,625	47,700	—	—	537,826	1123	—
Broilers	17,382	26,331	110,500	—	—	38,285	120	—
Unclassified/other	—	—	—	—	—	226,105	—	—
				Number			Percent	
Growers								
(plants & animals)	3,587	3,536	4,060	4,856	—	5,021	40	3

Numbers may not add due to rounding.

SOURCE: "Table 4.2: U.S. organic agriculture has expanded," in *Agricultural Fact Book 2000*, U.S. Department of Agriculture, Washington, D.C., 2000

Organic Agriculture

The National Organic Standards Board of the USDA defines organic agriculture in this manner:

Organic agriculture is an ecological production management system that promotes and enhances biodiversity, biological cycles and soil biological activity. It is based on minimal use of off-farm inputs and on management practices that restore, maintain and enhance ecological harmony. 'Organic' is a labeling term that denotes products produced under the authority of the Organic Foods Production Act. The principal guidelines for organic production are to use materials and practices that enhance the ecological balance of natural systems and that integrate the parts of the farming system into an ecological whole. Organic agriculture practices cannot ensure that products are completely free of residues; organic growing methods are used to minimize pollution from air, soil and water. Organic food handlers, processors and retailers adhere to standards that maintain the integrity of organic agriculture products. The primary goal of organic agriculture is to optimize the health and productivity of interdependent communities of soil life, plants, animals and people.

Organic farming became one of the fastest growing segments of U.S. agriculture during the 1990s. Certified organic cropland more than doubled in the United States during the 1990s, and several livestock sectors—dairy, eggs, and chicken—grew even faster. (See Table 1.2.) Farmers in 49 states dedicated 1.3 million acres of farmland to organic production. Idaho, California, North Dakota, Montana, and Minnesota were the top states in organic crop acreage. (See Figure 1.7.)

THE 1996 FARM ACT

The Federal Agriculture Improvement and Reform Act of 1996 (PL 104-127, also called the 1996 Farm Act) removes much of the former government control over what crops farmers are required to grow and how much is grown. Between 1973 and 1995, farmers were paid not to plant certain crops if there was a surplus of these crops. If crop prices dropped below specified levels, the federal government would make up the difference through "deficiency payments" to farmers.

The 1996 Farm Act changed income supports for eight major field crops—corn, sorghum, barley, oats, wheat, rice, upland cotton, and soybeans—by replacing the deficiency payments with a seven-year program of payments to ease farmers out of their reliance on price supports. These payments are fixed amounts that decrease over time until 2002.

BASELINE PROJECTIONS TO 2010

Crops, Livestock, and Poultry

Under provision of the 1996 Farm Act, farmers will be able to change their crops more easily because they will no longer be paid not to plant certain crops. However, they will be responsible for managing the risk of their choices. The *USDA Agricultural Baseline Projections to 2010* (Interagency Agricultural Projections Committee, USDA, Washington, D.C., 2000) presents projections for the agricultural sector from 2000 to 2010. The projections assume that the 1996 Farm Act will continue to be in force.

The USDA predicted that, overall, total acreage planted with the eight major field crops would rise

FIGURE 1.7

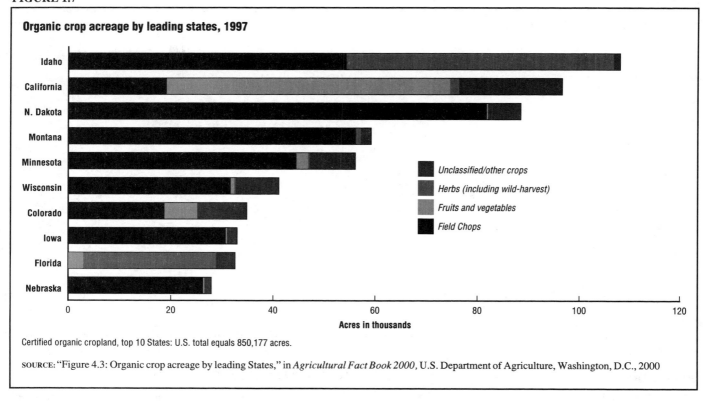

Organic crop acreage by leading states, 1997

Certified organic cropland, top 10 States: U.S. total equals 850,177 acres.

SOURCE: "Figure 4.3: Organic crop acreage by leading States," in *Agricultural Fact Book 2000,* U.S. Department of Agriculture, Washington, D.C., 2000

TABLE 1.3

Planted and harvested acreage for major field crops: baseline projections

	1999	2000	2001	2002	2003	2004	2005	2006	2007	2008	2009	2010
						Million acres						
Planted acreage, 8 major crops												
Corn	77.4	79.6	78.5	78.5	79.5	80.5	80.0	80.0	80.5	80.5	81.0	81.0
Sorghum	9.3	9.0	9.3	9.4	9.5	9.5	9.5	9.6	9.7	9.8	9.9	10.0
Barley	5.2	5.8	6.0	6.0	5.9	5.9	5.9	5.9	5.9	5.9	5.9	5.9
Oats	4.7	4.5	4.5	4.5	4.5	4.5	4.5	4.5	4.5	4.5	4.5	4.5
Wheat	62.7	62.5	62.0	61.0	62.5	63.5	64.5	64.5	64.5	65.0	65.5	66.0
Rice	3.5	3.1	3.2	3.2	3.2	3.2	3.1	3.1	3.1	3.1	3.1	3.0
Upland cotton	14.6	15.4	15.0	15.0	14.5	14.4	14.3	14.2	14.1	14.0	13.9	13.8
Soybeans	73.7	74.5	75.0	74.0	73.0	73.0	73.5	74.0	74.0	74.3	74.5	74.8
Total	251.1	254.4	253.5	251.6	252.6	254.5	255.3	255.8	256.3	257.0	258.3	259.0
Harvested acreage, 8 major crops												
Corn	70.5	73.0	71.7	71.7	72.7	73.7	73.2	73.2	73.7	73.7	74.2	74.2
Sorghum	8.5	7.7	8.3	8.4	8.5	8.5	8.5	8.6	8.7	8.8	8.9	9.0
Barley	4.7	5.2	5.5	5.5	5.4	5.4	5.4	5.4	5.4	5.4	5.4	5.4
Oats	2.5	2.3	2.3	2.3	2.3	2.3	2.3	2.3	2.3	2.3	2.3	2.3
Wheat	53.8	53.2	53.8	53.3	54.6	55.4	56.3	56.3	56.3	56.7	57.2	57.6
Rice	3.5	3.1	3.2	3.2	3.2	3.1	3.1	3.1	3.1	3.1	3.0	3.0
Upland cotton	13.1	13.4	13.8	13.8	13.3	13.2	13.2	13.1	13.0	12.9	12.8	12.7
Soybeans	72.4	73.0	74.0	73.0	72.0	72.0	72.5	73.0	73.0	73.3	73.5	73.8
Total	229.0	230.9	232.6	231.2	232.0	233.6	234.5	235.0	235.5	236.1	237.3	238.0

SOURCE: "Planted and harvested acreage for major field crops, baseline projections" in *USDA Agricultural Baseline Projections to 2010,* Economic Research Service, U.S. Department of Agriculture, Washington, D.C., February 2001

from 251 million acres in 1999 to 259 million acres in 2010, with much of the increase coming after 2002. Corn, wheat, sorghum, and soybeans would account for much of the growth. Total harvested acreage would parallel the acreage planted, staying flat through 2003 before going on an upward trend through 2010. (See Table 1.3.)

The USDA predicted that red meat consumption in the United States would gradually decrease from 124.8

TABLE 1.4

Per capita meat consumption: projections to 2010

Item	Units	1999	2000	2001	2002	2003	2004	2005	2006	2007	2008	2009	2010
Retail weight:													
Total beef	Pounds	69.1	69.7	66.0	65.0	64.1	63.4	63.1	64.0	64.8	64.9	64.5	64.3
Total veal	Pounds	0.7	0.7	0.6	0.6	0.6	0.6	0.5	0.5	0.5	0.5	0.4	0.4
Total pork	Pounds	53.9	52.4	53.2	55.6	54.3	53.3	52.9	52.6	52.3	51.9	51.4	51.1
Lamb and mutton	Pounds	1.2	1.1	1.1	1.1	1.0	1.0	1.0	1.0	1.0	1.0	0.9	0.9
Total red meat	Pounds	124.8	123.8	120.9	122.2	120.0	118.3	117.6	118.1	118.6	118.2	117.4	116.7
Broilers	Pounds	77.9	78.7	81.3	83.3	85.1	86.8	88.6	90.2	91.5	92.6	93.9	95.0
Other chicken	Pounds	0.6	0.9	0.9	0.9	0.9	0.9	0.8	0.8	0.8	0.8	0.8	0.8
Turkeys	Pounds	18.0	18.1	18.2	18.7	18.8	19.0	19.0	19.0	18.9	18.7	18.5	18.3
Total poultry	Pounds	96.4	97.7	100.4	102.8	104.8	106.7	108.4	110.0	111.2	112.1	113.2	114.1
Red meat & poultry	Pounds	221.2	221.6	221.4	225.0	224.9	225.0	225.9	228.1	229.8	230.4	230.5	230.8
Boneless weight:													
Total beef	Pounds	65.4	66.0	62.5	61.5	60.7	60.1	59.8	60.6	61.4	61.5	61.1	60.9
Total veal	Pounds	0.6	0.6	0.5	0.5	0.5	0.5	0.4	0.4	0.4	0.4	0.4	0.4
Total pork	Pounds	50.6	49.2	50.0	52.2	51.0	50.1	49.7	49.4	49.2	48.8	48.3	48.0
Lamb & mutton	Pounds	0.9	0.8	0.8	0.8	0.8	0.7	0.7	0.7	0.7	0.7	0.7	0.7
Total red meat	Pounds	117.5	116.6	113.8	115.0	113.0	111.4	110.7	111.2	111.7	111.3	110.5	109.9
Broilers	Pounds	55.1	55.7	57.6	58.9	60.2	61.4	62.7	63.8	64.8	65.6	66.4	67.2
Other chicken	Pounds	0.4	0.6	0.6	0.6	0.6	0.6	0.5	0.5	0.5	0.5	0.5	0.5
Turkeys	Pounds	14.2	14.3	14.4	14.8	14.9	15.0	15.0	15.0	14.9	14.8	14.6	14.5
Total poultry	Pounds	69.7	70.6	72.5	74.2	75.7	77.0	78.2	79.3	80.2	80.8	81.5	82.2
Red meat and poultry	Pounds	187.1	187.1	186.3	189.2	188.6	188.4	188.9	190.5	191.9	192.1	192.0	192.1

SOURCE: "Per capita meat consumption, retail and boneless weight" in *USDA Agricultural Baseline Projections to 2010,* Economic Research Service, U.S. Department of Agriculture, Washington, D.C., February 2001

TABLE 1.5

Consumer expenditures for meat

Item	1999	2000	2001	2002	2003	2004	2005	2006	2007	2008	2009	2010
Beef, dollars per person	198.98	212.43	204.63	202.89	205.86	208.63	210.82	212.58	214.51	217.63	221.21	224.51
Percent of income	0.82	0.83	0.76	0.72	0.70	0.67	0.65	0.62	0.60	0.58	0.57	0.55
Percent of meat expenditures	42.63	43.51	42.06	41.82	41.56	41.32	41.13	41.14	41.17	41.09	40.90	40.73
Pork, dollars per person	129.78	135.23	137.33	135.80	137.23	138.50	139.33	139.22	139.09	139.78	140.89	141.71
Percent of income	0.53	0.53	0.51	0.48	0.46	0.45	0.43	0.41	0.39	0.37	0.36	0.35
Percent of meat expenditures	27.80	27.70	28.23	27.99	27.71	27.43	27.18	26.95	26.70	26.39	26.05	25.71
Broilers, dollars per person	120.22	121.95	125.99	128.12	133.79	139.30	144.16	147.09	150.09	155.22	161.81	168.22
Percent of income	0.49	0.47	0.47	0.45	0.45	0.45	0.44	0.43	0.42	0.42	0.41	0.41
Percent of meat expenditures	25.75	24.98	25.90	26.41	27.01	27.59	28.12	28.47	28.81	29.31	29.92	30.51
Turkeys, dollars per person	17.83	18.59	18.58	18.36	18.44	18.46	18.30	17.79	17.29	17.05	16.95	16.84
Percent of income	0.07	0.07	0.07	0.06	0.06	0.06	0.06	0.05	0.05	0.05	0.04	0.04
Percent of meat expenditures	3.82	3.81	3.82	3.78	3.72	3.66	3.57	3.44	3.32	3.22	3.13	3.06
Total meat, dollars per person	466.81	488.20	486.53	485.18	495.32	504.89	512.61	516.67	520.98	529.68	540.85	551.29
Percent of income	1.92	1.90	1.80	1.72	1.67	1.63	1.58	1.52	1.46	1.42	1.39	1.35

SOURCE: "Consumer expenditures for meats" in *USDA Agricultural Baseline Projections to 2010,* Economic Research Service, U.S. Department of Agriculture, Washington, D.C., February 2001

pounds per person in 1999 to 116.7 in 2010. Poultry consumption, on the other hand, is expected to increase substantially over the same period from 96.4 pounds to 114.1 pounds. (See Table 1.4.)

In 1999 consumers spent 42.6 percent of their meat expenditures on beef; by 2010 this is expected to drop to 40.7 percent. The per capita expenditure, however, would increase, from about $199 to $224. On the other hand, the percentage of expenditures on chicken (broilers) is expected to rise from 25.8 percent to 30.5 percent over the

same period, while per capita dollars rise sharply from $120 to $168. (See Table 1.5.) The USDA attributes the poultry increase to lower production costs and prices, compared to other meats, but consumer interest in lower-fat diets might also play a role.

Farm Income

Net farm income was $40 billion in 2000, down from nearly $55 billion in 1996. This largely reflected a reduction in direct government payments. The USDA projects

FIGURE 1.8

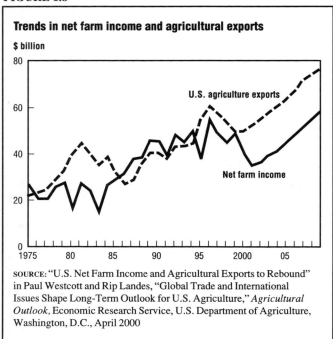

Trends in net farm income and agricultural exports

$ billion

U.S. agriculture exports

Net farm income

SOURCE: "U.S. Net Farm Income and Agricultural Exports to Rebound" in Paul Westcott and Rip Landes, "Global Trade and International Issues Shape Long-Term Outlook for U.S. Agriculture," *Agricultural Outlook,* Economic Research Service, U.S. Department of Agriculture, Washington, D.C., April 2000

that income will rise to nearly $50 billion by 2005 and to $60 billion in 2010 and beyond. (See Figure 1.8.) Nonetheless, farm income gains (2 percent annually) will be less than inflation gains (2.7 percent annually); therefore, the real value of net farm income is expected to decline throughout the period of 2000 to 2010.

CHAPTER 2
WHAT DO AMERICANS EAT?

Over the past 20 years, Americans have slowly changed their eating habits. While earlier generations grew up eating meat, potatoes, and Mom's apple pie, food purchasers today are often choosing convenience foods and foods away from home. Many Americans are aware that there is a direct link between diet and disease. Cholesterol can clog arteries, causing cardiovascular disease and eventual heart attack, the number one killer in America. Americans consumed less red meat and more poultry and fish in the 1990s than in the 1980s. And while Americans are eating more grains, they still do not eat as many whole-grain products, legumes, vegetables, or fruits as recommended by the federal *Dietary Guidelines for Americans*. In addition, Americans are eating more foods with large amounts of refined sugars.

FOOD INTAKE

Over 5,100 people nationwide participated in the 1996 U.S. Department of Agriculture (USDA) *Continuing Survey of Food Intakes by Individuals (CSFII), popularly known as the What We Eat in America Survey* (Agricultural Research Service, Beltsville, Maryland, 1997), the U.S. government's main source of data on individual food intakes. Participants tracked their food intake for two non-consecutive days, and 1,920 of those 20 years old and older answered questions on their attitudes and knowledge about dietary guidance and health. The responses of the latter group were recorded in the *Diet and Health Knowledge Survey* (Agricultural Research Service, Beltsville, Maryland, 1997).

Red Meat, Poultry, and Fish

The CSFII found that most Americans (85.7 percent) eat meat, poultry, or fish on a given day. Frankfurters, sausages, and luncheon meats, as well as mixtures of meat, poultry, and fish (for example, casserole, meat loaf, corn dog, tuna salad, chicken soup, and sandwiches such as

cheeseburgers) were the most popular forms of meat. An almost equal proportion of participants reported eating beef (19.7 percent) and poultry (21.7 percent). (See Table 2.1.)

Meat becomes part of the American diet at an early age. While almost 30 percent of babies under one year old ate meat (refers to total kinds of meat), by the time they reached the age of 1 to 2 years, 4 out of 5 (80 percent) were eating meat. Among adults, young women between the ages of 12 and 29 were less likely to eat meat, although 4 out of 5 still ate meat (See Table 2.1. Note: The data tables for percentages of individuals who ate particular foods were based on day one of the survey).

Grain Products

Nearly everyone (96.7 percent) had eaten some grain products during day one of the survey. Yeast breads and rolls were the most popular grain products, consumed by two-thirds (65.9 percent) of all individuals, followed by cereals and pasta, eaten by nearly half (46.8 percent) of all survey participants. Cakes, cookies, and other pastries were nearly as popular, indulged in by 41.9 percent of participants. (See Table 2.2.)

Fruits and Vegetables

Although nutritionists encourage people to eat fruits for a healthy diet, the survey revealed that many people do not follow this advice. Overall, little more than half the participants (52.6 percent) reported eating fruits. About one-fifth (20.1 percent) consumed their citrus fruits in the forms of juices, and about 13 percent had eaten an apple or a banana. Young children and those over 60 were more likely to have eaten apples and bananas. (See Table 2.3.)

While 82.7 percent of individuals ate vegetables, the primary choice was potatoes (45.6 percent), with 28.5 percent choosing fried potatoes, usually French fries. The next most popular vegetables were tomatoes (39.9 percent), which, in addition to fresh, were ingested in various

TABLE 2.1

Percent of individuals consuming various types of meat over the course of one day, by sex and age, 1996

Sex and age (years)	Percentage of population	Total	Beef	Pork	Lamb, veal, game	Organ meats	Frankfurters, sausages, luncheon meats	Poultry Total	Poultry Chicken	Fish and shellfish	Mixtures mainly meat, poultry, fish
	Percent						Percent				
Males and females:											
Under 1	1.1	29.9	1.7†	1.7†	0.0†	0.0†	3.2†	6.2†	5.4†	2.6†	18.6
1–2	3.0	80.2	12.5	7.4	.9†	0.0†	27.1	24.5	22.1	5.1	37.2
3–5	4.7	85.5	15.8	13.0	1.2†	.1†	33.5	26.5	24.9	6.9	30.1
5 and under	8.8	76.5	12.8	9.6	1.0†	.1†	27.4	23.2	21.5	5.7	31.0
Males:											
6–11	4.6	84.3	21.5	12.6	.6†	0.0†	28.5	20.0	18.9	3.0†	40.0
12–19	5.9	87.8	25.9	15.5	.6†	0.0†	39.9	19.6	18.6	4.5	38.0
20–29	7.2	89.6	23.4	16.1	.9†	0.0†	27.9	23.4	17.9	7.6	39.8
30–39	8.1	90.6	26.1	17.2	1.3†	.1†	32.3	18.1	15.4	10.1	42.9
40–49	7.0	88.9	28.7	16.3	.4†	.3†	33.7	22.5	19.4	10.1	39.4
50–59	4.7	91.3	24.1	20.8	1.1†	.7†	33.6	17.7	13.0	16.3	34.7
60–69	3.4	90.8	23.0	18.3	1.6†	.4†	34.6	19.6	15.3	12.9	37.7
70 and over	3.4	92.1	20.8	27.1	1.6†	.4†	34.1	18.2	16.7	11.5	34.0
20 and over	33.9	90.3	25.0	18.4	1.0†	.3†	32.3	20.2	16.6	10.9	39.0
Females:											
6–11	4.4	84.3	14.8	9.3	.2†	.3†	27.2	26.5	23.8	5.9	37.1
12–19	5.6	81.1	19.4	11.0	0.0†	0.0†	26.4	25.0	22.8	5.0	34.5
20–29	6.9	77.7	14.8	11.2	.3†	.3†	22.7	18.7	17.8	6.5	39.7
30–39	8.6	83.9	15.6	15.9	.4†	0.0†	29.8	22.3	19.5	6.7	38.1
40–49	7.2	86.4	15.9	19.8	1.1†	0.0†	23.1	22.6	17.9	10.1	34.7
50–59	5.1	86.1	14.6	17.8	1.2†	.9†	20.7	25.9	19.5	12.3	39.2
60–69	3.9	87.1	16.7	14.3	1.8†	0.0†	29.0	20.7	18.5	11.0	34.9
70 and over	5.1	87.9	18.6	26.4	.5†	.9†	20.6	23.2	21.4	11.1	27.8
20 and over	36.8	84.4	15.9	17.3	.8	.3†	24.6	22.1	19.0	9.2	36.1
All individuals	100.0	85.7	19.7	16.0	.8	.2	28.7	21.7	18.8	8.5	36.9

†Estimates based on small cell sizes may tend to be less statistically reliable than estimates based on larger cell sizes. Cell size refers to the unweighted number of individuals in a given sex-age group or demographic group.
Note: Excludes breast-fed children.

SOURCE: "Meat, poultry, and fish: Percentages of individuals consuming foods from various food groups, by sex and age, 1 day, 1996" in *Results From USDA's 1996 Continuing Survey of Food Intakes by Individuals and 1996 Diet and Health Knowledge Survey*, U.S. Agricultural Research Service, Beltsville, MD, 1997

forms—tomato juice; ketchup, salsa, chili sauce, and other tomato sauces; and other mixtures with tomatoes as a main ingredient, such as tomato-based soup. (See Table 2.4.)

Milk and Milk Products

Whole milk has a high fat content that is generally not considered desirable; experts advise drinking skim (fat-free) milk instead. The survey found that many consumers had switched to low-fat milk (25.4 percent, which includes reduced-fat and low-fat milk) but were not as enthusiastic about skim milk (11.5 percent). One-third (33 percent) ate cheese, and 16.1 percent ate milk desserts, primarily ice cream. (See Table 2.5.)

Beverages and Miscellaneous Foods

Carbonated soft drinks were the most popular beverage, consumed by half (50.3 percent) of the participants, although coffee was more popular with those 20 years old and over (54.2 percent). Over one-fifth (22.5 percent) of men 20 years and older drank an alcoholic beverage, compared to 12.1 percent of women 20 years and older. Twice

as many children (40.4 percent) ages 3 to 5 consumed fruit drinks and -ades, compared to 21.2 percent (Table 2.3) of the same age group who consumed citrus fruit juices. Overall, about one-third of children ages 1 to 11 drank fruit drinks and -ades. (See Table 2.6.)

Over half (54.1 percent) of those surveyed consumed fats and oils, which included vegetable oils, table and cooking fats, salad dressings, nondairy cream substitutes, tartar sauce, and other sauces that were mainly fat or oil. Half (52.3 percent) consumed sugars and sweets, which included sweet sauces, gelatin desserts, jellies, jams, preserves, and candies. About one-fifth (19.1 percent) ate eggs. (See Table 2.7.)

PER CAPITA FOOD CONSUMPTION

The USDA Economic Research Service (ERS) tracks the annual per capita (per person) food consumption by Americans in its food supply series *Food Consumption, Prices, and Expenditures*. The ERS calculates the amount of food available for human consumption by subtracting

TABLE 2.2

Percent of individuals consuming various types of grain products over the course of one day, by sex and age, 1996

Sex and age (years)	Percentage of population	Total	Yeast breads and rolls	Cereals and pasta Total	Ready-to-eat cereals	Rice	Pasta	Quick breads, pancakes, french toast	Cakes, cookies, pastries, pies	Crackers, popcorn, pretzels, corn chips	Mixtures mainly grain
	Percent					Percent					
Males and females:											
Under 1	1.1	74.4	10.3†	65.5	6.0†	.9†	2.0†	6.2†	16.5	8.0†	13.7
1–2	3.0	98.7†	53.5	70.5	46.5	13.5	11.7	27.3	44.9	32.8	41.8
3–5	4.7	99.4†	63.4	66.5	50.1	10.5	9.8	27.1	46.5	39.0	48.1
5 and under	8.8	95.9	53.2	67.7	43.2	10.3	9.4	24.4	42.1	32.9	41.5
Males:											
6–11	4.6	98.2†	57.9	56.1	46.8	8.0	7.0	27.4	51.7	32.1	41.6
12–19	5.9	97.8†	64.5	49.8	34.8	11.7	9.3	23.3	44.3	29.1	51.8
20–29	7.2	93.7	57.9	35.4	15.9	11.5	9.1	22.4	30.0	27.3	40.1
30–39	8.1	93.7	65.9	37.2	22.3	11.5	7.3	23.9	37.9	26.1	35.8
40–49	7.0	96.3†	70.0	45.3	21.1	13.9	11.1	21.6	45.7	22.5	34.5
50–59	4.7	97.8†	72.0	39.1	21.7	12.2	7.2	25.7	40.5	29.3	31.1
60–69	3.4	97.9†	79.7	51.7	29.6	11.2	7.5	23.6	38.1	23.3	24.1
70 and over	3.4	97.6†	79.1	58.8	38.9	4.8†	4.7†	20.7	52.9	25.6	20.2
20 and over	33.9	95.6	68.6	42.4	23.0	11.4	8.2	23.0	39.7	25.7	33.1
Females:											
6–11	4.4	99.4†	65.8	59.5	43.6	8.6	9.2	26.9	51.7	35.8	43.7
12–19	5.6	97.4†	62.8	47.4	30.1	8.4	10.1	19.1	40.7	25.6	44.3
20–29	6.9	97.3†	62.8	41.6	25.1	10.5	6.8	19.5	39.6	26.8	42.5
30–39	8.6	95.4	64.1	38.2	23.1	8.2	9.4	23.4	37.8	31.1	38.6
40–49	7.2	97.0†	69.4	43.3	21.0	15.1	8.3	20.4	40.6	26.7	32.4
50–59	5.1	98.3†	70.7	39.7	18.6	11.6	6.9	26.6	37.6	24.5	28.9
60–69	3.9	97.2†	73.0	42.5	24.6	8.3	8.5	20.1	42.8	27.2	20.2
70 and over	5.1	98.3†	75.2	52.6	31.8	4.5†	3.0†	25.9	52.9	20.4	17.4
20 and over	36.8	97.1	68.3	42.5	23.8	10.0	7.4	22.5	41.3	26.6	31.9
All individuals	100.0	96.7	65.9	46.8	28.2	10.3	8.2	23.1	41.9	27.6	36.0

†Estimates based on small cell sizes may tend to be less statistically reliable than estimates based on larger cell sizes. Cell size refers to the unweighted number of individuals in a given sex-age group or demographic group.

Note: Excludes breast-fed children.

SOURCE: "Grain products: Percentages of individuals consuming foods from various food groups, by sex and age, 1 day, 1996" in *Results From USDA's 1996 Continuing Survey of Food Intakes by Individuals and 1996 Diet and Health Knowledge Survey*, U.S. Agricultural Research Service, Beltsville, MD, 1997

measurable uses (exports; seed, feed, and industrial use; and end-of-year inventories) from the total food supply (food produced, imports, and beginning inventories). (See Figure 2.1.) The per capita consumption is then calculated by dividing the food available for human consumption (also referred to as "food disappearance") by the U.S. total population, including the armed forces overseas.

Food disappearance is not an accurate measure of how much food is eaten, but an indicator of trends in consumption over time. ERS data do not reflect how much food is purchased and then wasted, how much is fed to pets, or how much fish and game are obtained by consumers without purchasing them. The data also include unknown amounts of foods used as ingredients in processed foods that are exported.

In the last 30 years, the consumption patterns of Americans have undergone some changes. Factors that are responsible for these changes include:

- The introduction of convenience foods and the growth of the away-from-home food market.

- Advances in food enrichment and fortification.

- Improved nutrition labeling.

- The continuing public education on the correlation of diet and health.

- Sociodemographic trends, such as the rise in single-parent and two-earner households, the growing numbers of working women, an aging population, and increased racial and ethnic diversity.

Red Meat, Poultry, and Fish

In 1998, while continuing to consume plenty of red meat (beef, pork, veal, lamb, and mutton), more Americans chose leaner meat. The average American consumed a total of 195.4 pounds of red meat, poultry, and fish (boneless, trimmed-weight equivalent), 16 pounds above the 1980 level. However, the per person consumption of red meat was lower—on average, each person consumed 11 pounds less red meat than in 1980. Each person consumed 25 pounds more poultry than in 1980 and over 2 pounds more fish and shellfish, although fish has yet to become a major part of the American diet. (See Table 2.8.)

TABLE 2.3

Percent of individuals consuming various types of fruit over the course of one day, by sex and age, 1996

Sex and age (years)	Percentage of population	Total	Citrus fruits and juices		Dried fruits	Other fruits, mixtures, and juices					
			Total	Juices		Total	Apples	Bananas	Melons and berries	Other fruits and mixtures mainly fruit	Noncitrus juices and nectars
	Percent					Percent					
Males and females:											
Under 1	1.1	63.4	1.9†	.5†	0.0†	62.9	19.5	11.8	1.6†	39.7	32.2
1–2	3.0	79.4	28.8	21.8	5.4	68.0	23.2	22.8	7.8	23.4	40.3
3–5	4.7	65.7	26.3	21.2	3.9	54.8	17.7	13.7	6.3	16.9	26.2
5 and under	8.8	70.1	24.0	18.7	3.9	60.3	19.8	16.6	6.2	22.0	31.7
Males:											
6–11	4.6	47.5	18.5	16.1	.4†	39.8	18.0	7.0	6.5	11.8	9.5
12–19	5.9	42.1	23.6	18.3	1.1†	26.3	7.6	5.6	5.0	8.9	7.4
20–29	7.2	39.0	21.2	19.4	.5†	25.1	6.4	7.9	4.7	9.0	3.0†
30–39	8.1	36.9	20.3	16.9	1.2†	21.9	5.1	8.8	4.9	7.5	3.7
40–49	7.0	47.6	25.3	19.4	1.8†	31.9	10.4	12.0	6.0	11.5	5.6
50–59	4.7	56.5	31.2	23.6	2.3†	42.5	13.7	20.5	7.3	13.2	5.9
60–69	3.4	64.8	34.1	25.7	4.7	49.6	15.1	25.8	11.0	14.5	4.6
70 and over	3.4	67.3	34.7	28.5	6.9	53.5	19.9	28.2	13.3	20.8	5.5
20 and over	33.9	48.2	25.9	20.9	2.2	33.5	10.2	14.6	6.9	11.5	4.5
Females:											
6–11	4.4	62.0	25.5	18.2	1.2†	47.5	15.7	7.2	6.6	19.5	14.7
12–19	5.6	44.6	23.6	19.5	1.3†	29.9	11.3	6.0	5.5	9.2	9.3
20–29	6.9	47.6	28.5	21.6	.8†	31.6	10.1	11.5	4.5	10.0	6.2
30–39	8.6	47.6	20.9	16.2	3.5†	34.2	9.1	13.7	10.5	11.7	4.2
40–49	7.2	49.6	22.6	16.2	1.2†	37.8	12.3	13.1	9.7	12.6	5.4
50–59	5.1	61.5	33.5	23.5	3.1†	48.4	14.9	20.6	11.5	13.9	3.2†
60–69	3.9	66.1	32.7	22.5	4.3†	52.2	15.5	24.4	14.8	18.1	5.3
70 and over	5.1	69.9	36.7	29.3	5.8†	56.6	12.7	25.6	9.0	22.3	5.6†
20 and over	36.8	55.0	27.8	20.7	2.9	41.4	11.9	16.9	9.6	14.0	5.0
All individuals	100.0	52.6	25.8	20.1	2.4	39.1	12.2	13.9	7.6	13.4	8.2

†Estimates based on small cell sizes may tend to be less statistically reliable than estimates based on larger cell sizes. Cell size refers to the unweighted number of individuals in a given sex-age group or demographic group.

Note: Excludes brest-fed children.

SOURCE: "Fruits: Percentages of individuals consuming foods from various food groups, by sex and age, 1 day, 1996" in *Results From USDA's 1996 Continuing Survey of Food Intakes by Individuals and 1996 Diet and Health Knowledge Survey*, U.S. Agricultural Research Service, Beltsville, MD, 1997

Concerns about fat and cholesterol have led to the production of leaner meat, the practice of trimming outside fat before retail sale, and the introduction of processed meat products with lower fat contents. In the 1990s, despite high per capita total meat consumption, red meat, particularly beef, contributed less and poultry contributed more to the per capita food consumption. (See Figure 2.2 and Figure 2.3.)

Health concerns relating to beef consumption have helped boost the sale of poultry. The poultry industry responded to consumer demand by introducing new products, including boneless, skinless chicken and turkey; chicken and turkey franks, sausages, and deli meats; and ground chicken and turkey.

The growing numbers of working women and single-parent families have influenced meat consumption. Hamburger, which can be prepared quickly, accounted for 40 percent of the beef consumed in 1995, compared to 26 percent in 1970. Roasts, which require longer preparation time, experienced a sharp decline in sales. In addition Americans now eat out more often, especially in fast-food restaurants that feature hamburgers, chicken, and pizza. Since 1980, as the total per capita consumption of chicken has climbed rapidly, the share provided by food-service establishments almost doubled from 25 percent in 1970 to 46 percent in 1996.

Flour and Cereal Products

In 1997 per capita use of flour and cereal products totaled 197 pounds, a 50 percent increase since 1972 but still about 100 pounds below the 1909 level of 300 pounds per person. (At the beginning of the twentieth century, grain products were the major source of protein in the American diet.) (See Figure 2.4 and Figure 2.5.) The USDA attributes the increase in flour and grain use to a greater appreciation for variety breads and other in-store bakery items and to the fast-food sales of hamburger buns, other sandwich rolls, pizza dough, and tortillas. The popularity of ethnic foods, especially Mexican foods, has been responsible in part for the increased per capita consumption of flour and grains.

Wheat is the major grain product consumed in the United States. The per capita use of wheat has risen 26

TABLE 2.4

Percent of individuals consuming various types of vegetables over the course of one day, by sex and age, 1996

Sex and age (years)	Percentage of population	Total	White potatoes Total	White potatoes Fried	Dark-green vegetables	Deep-yellow vegetables	Tomatoes	Lettuce, lettuce-based salads	Green beans	Corn, green peas, lima beans	Other vegetables
	Percent						Percent				
Males and females:											
Under 1	1.1	52.7	13.9	5.2†	3.6†	20.8	.6†	0.0†	15.5	9.4†	14.4
1–2	3.0	74.4	40.5	25.1	7.0	11.7	26.2	5.8	11.0	17.6	20.1
3–5	4.7	73.3	46.5	34.2	6.2	9.9	33.2	9.2	7.5	14.2	22.4
5 and under	8.8	71.0	40.3	27.4	6.2	11.9	26.6	6.9	9.7	14.7	20.6
Males:											
6–11	4.6	76.8	51.6	38.7	8.2	7.9	34.2	15.2	7.6	16.4	26.6
12–19	5.9	80.8	48.9	35.8	2.1†	9.4	45.7	27.9	3.7†	6.1	33.2
20–29	7.2	82.6	50.4	36.8	7.0	6.8	47.3	24.0	3.4†	7.0	38.1
30–39	8.1	87.9	50.1	34.2	9.9	10.7	42.7	26.4	6.3	10.9	52.7
40–49	7.0	86.9	46.2	29.1	8.6	13.9	39.7	27.5	7.5	15.5	52.1
50–59	4.7	90.8	47.5	25.2	11.6	15.9	46.6	32.3	6.7	17.3	48.9
60–69	3.4	85.1	43.0	18.9	16.2	20.3	43.9	29.4	8.8	12.3	52.8
70 and over	3.4	83.8	46.9	13.8	13.1	18.6	36.1	27.3	12.3	16.6	50.1
20 and over	33.9	86.3	48.0	28.8	10.2	13.0	43.0	27.3	6.8	12.6	48.7
Females:											
6–11	4.4	83.7	54.5	43.6	3.9†	14.1	35.6	17.7	6.5	16.9	30.5
12–19	5.6	84.0	49.6	41.7	14.1	13.1	41.6	30.6	3.2†	5.4	38.4
20–29	6.9	79.6	41.4	25.8	8.0	11.3	42.7	25.3	5.9	5.3	41.3
30–39	8.6	85.3	47.1	26.6	13.4	15.7	39.7	31.0	4.5	12.3	46.3
40–49	7.2	82.1	40.1	23.1	12.0	16.7	37.7	33.5	6.2	10.7	43.3
50–59	5.1	82.5	40.3	20.1	14.9	15.6	42.9	32.2	8.2	10.1	48.1
60–69	3.9	82.3	36.8	14.9	13.9	14.4	41.0	29.7	9.8	9.2	50.0
70 and over	5.1	85.7	41.7	15.5	11.8	10.7	38.8	25.0	8.7	15.5	51.6
20 and over	36.8	82.9	41.9	22.1	12.2	14.2	40.3	29.6	6.8	10.5	46.2
All individuals	100.0	82.7	45.6	28.5	9.9	13.0	39.9	25.6	6.7	11.6	42.0

†Estimates based on small cell sizes may tend to be less statistically reliable than estimates based on larger cell sizes. Cell size refers to the unweighted number of individuals in a given sex-age group or demographic group.

Note: Excludes breast-fed children.

SOURCE: "Vegetables: Percentages of individuals consuming foods from various food groups, by sex and age, 1 day, 1996" in *Results From USDA's 1996 Continuing Survey of Food Intakes by Individuals and 1996 Diet and Health Knowledge Survey*, U.S. Agricultural Research Service, Beltsville, MD, 1997

percent since 1980. As rice, corn products, and oat products have gained popularity, however, wheat's share of total grain consumption has declined. (See Table 2.8.)

Between 1980 and 1997 consumption of breakfast cereals increased 41 percent—from 12 pounds to 16.9 pounds per capita, even though cereal prices have risen faster than the prices for most other grocery foods. (See Table 2.8.) Consumers' goal of increasing the fiber in their diets, the convenience of serving cereals for breakfast, and advertising touting the health benefits of cereal have contributed to this increase.

Fruits and Vegetables

Total per capita use of fruits and vegetables reached 710.8 pounds in 1997, up 19 percent from 1982. (See Figure 2.6.) Much of this increase occurred since 1982, the year the landmark report *Diet, Nutrition, and Cancer* (National Academy of Sciences [NAS], Washington, D.C., 1982) was published. In the report, a panel of expert scientists assembled by the NAS stressed the beneficial effects of fruits, vegetables, and whole-grain products on overall health. They also reported on the likelihood that these foods might help reduce the risk of cancer. The panel suggested using citrus fruits, vegetables in the cabbage family, and vegetables and fruits rich in carotene.

Dairy Products

In 1998 Americans drank an average of 14.8 percent less milk than in 1980. Between 1980 and 1998, Americans decreased their average consumption of whole milk by 50 percent (from 16.5 to 8.0 gallons per capita), while increasing by 50 percent their low-fat and skim milk consumption (from 9.4 to 14.1 gallons per capita). (See Table 2.8 and Figure 2.7.) The USDA attributes these diet changes to concerns about cholesterol and fat, the declining numbers of teenage males, an increasing milk-sugar (lactose) intolerance due to the growing ethnic diversity in the country, and the growing preference for soft drinks. However, while consumers cut back on whole milk, they increased their use of fluid cream products—half-and-half, light and heavy cream, sour cream, eggnog, and dips—from 10.5 to 17.3 pounds. (See Table 2.8.)

The consumption of cheese continued to rise, increasing 62 percent between 1980 and 1998, from 17.5 to 28.4

TABLE 2.5

Percent of individuals consuming various types of milk and milk products over the course of one day, by sex and age, 1996

Sex and age (years)	Percentage of population	Total	Milk, milk drinks, yogurt Total	Fluid milk Total	Whole	Low fat	Skim	Yogurt	Milk desserts	Cheese
	Percent					Percent				
Males and females:										
Under 1	1.1	82.9	82.9	8.6†	4.8†	1.3†	0.0†	1.0†	13.7	4.8†
1–2	3.0	95.3	91.6	87.3	54.8	32.0	2.6†	8.8	13.0	32.0
3–5	4.7	92.9	85.6	82.5	40.8	39.4	6.8	5.4	21.8	35.4
5 and under	8.8	92.4	87.3	74.6	40.9	32.0	4.5	6.0	17.8	30.3
Males:										
6–11	4.6	90.1	80.6	75.5	28.5	43.4	8.0	2.6†	29.1	28.0
12–19	5.9	82.1	67.4	61.0	20.9	30.5	10.7	2.2†	12.8	40.8
20–29	7.2	70.1	44.0	40.0	12.9	19.5	8.4	3.8	10.3	36.8
30–39	8.1	73.8	50.7	46.7	18.7	20.3	7.7	3.3	14.0	40.8
40–49	7.0	71.7	50.4	47.4	14.8	20.2	12.5	4.2	12.2	30.9
50–59	4.7	73.0	52.6	50.3	11.0	26.7	12.6	2.0†	18.8	28.5
60–69	3.4	79.6	64.9	61.7	16.5	28.0	17.2	2.3†	20.9	29.9
70 and over	3.4	84.1	69.0	66.9	21.3	29.4	20.2	.8†	27.3	28.0
20 and over	33.9	74.1	52.7	49.5	15.6	22.7	11.7	3.1	15.5	33.8
Females:										
6–11	4.4	89.4	84.1	78.3	37.5	37.5	6.5	.9†	20.3	23.8
12–19	5.6	74.9	49.8	45.5	17.3	21.4	8.2	1.3†	15.0	38.5
20–29	6.9	71.5	50.6	45.8	17.2	16.8	12.4	2.9†	9.1	33.2
30–39	8.6	76.9	54.0	49.7	15.6	23.1	10.7	7.2	13.9	39.0
40–49	7.2	75.3	50.3	46.8	14.8	22.1	11.7	5.6	11.9	38.4
50–59	5.1	79.1	59.3	50.5	8.7	21.4	19.7	9.2	19.8	27.2
60–69	3.9	76.1	56.6	53.6	11.5	21.4	21.5	5.6	16.7	29.3
70 and over	5.1	83.0	66.6	63.2	16.4	30.8	17.5	4.9†	22.4	19.8
20 and over	36.8	76.6	55.4	50.8	14.5	22.4	14.5	5.9	14.9	32.5
All individuals	100.0	78.6	60.1	55.1	19.4	25.4	11.5	4.1	16.1	33.0

†Estimates based on small cell sizes may tend to be less statistically reliable than estimates based on larger cell sizes. Cell size refers to the unweighted number of individuals in a given sex-age group or demographic group.

Note: Excludes breast-fed children.

SOURCE: "Milk and milk products: Percentages of individuals consuming foods from various food groups, by sex and age, 1 day, 1996" in *Results From USDA's 1996 Continuing Survey of Food Intakes by Individuals and 1996 Diet and Health Knowledge Survey,* U.S. Agricultural Research Service, Beltsville, MD, 1997

pounds per person. (See Table 2.8 and Figure 2.8.) The continuing growth in cheese consumption may be due to the proliferation of convenience food—two-thirds of cheese comes in commercially manufactured and prepared foods, such as pizzas, tacos, fast-food sandwiches, and packaged snack foods. Cheese is also offered in salad bars and in sauces for various vegetables, such as baked potatoes. New cheese products (in convenient resealable containers), including cheese blends for the preparation of ethnic dishes, have also contributed to the increased per capita use.

From 1980 to 1998, the consumption of cheddar cheese rose 39 percent, from 6.9 to 9.6 pounds per capita. The use of Italian cheeses increased threefold over the same time period, from 4.4 to 11.3 pounds. Per capita consumption of mozzarella cheese, the main pizza cheese, also rose from 3.0 pounds in 1980 to 8.7 pounds per capita in 1998.

Eggs

In 1998 each American, on average, consumed 244 eggs, a 10 percent decrease from 271 eggs in 1980. (See Table 2.8.) Since the 1980s, eggs have been consumed not only as shell eggs but also as egg products (processed eggs that are sold to food manufacturers and food-service operators). Consumers use them as liquid eggs, which are sold in food stores. These liquid eggs are generally made from egg whites and are used as noncholesterol substitutes for shell eggs. Consumers also use egg products as ingredients in processed foods and food-service menu items; for example, cake mixes, pasta, and baked goods. The decline in egg use seems to have leveled. Recently nutritionists have been recommending limited use of eggs rather than eliminating them from the diet completely.

Fats and Oils

Despite the growing health concerns about fats and oils, Americans consumed 8.4 pounds more fats and oils per person in 1998 than in 1980, up from 56.9 to 65.3 pounds. (See Table 2.8 and Figure 2.9.) This increase is probably due to the increased consumption of fried foods in restaurants and the increased use of salad dressings. According to the USDA, the average woman 19 to 50 years old gets more fat from salad dressings than from any other food.

TABLE 2.6

Percent of individuals consuming various types of beverages over the course of one day, by sex and age, 1996

Sex and age (years)	Percentage of population	Total	Alcoholic Total	Wine	Beer and ale	Nonalcoholic Total	Coffee	Tea	Fruit drinks and -ades Total	Regular	Low calorie	Carbonated soft drinks Total	Regular	Low calorie
	Percent							Percent						
Males and females:														
Under 1	1.1	8.0†	0.0†	0.0†	0.0†	8.0†	0.0†	.7†	7.3†	4.3†	2.4†	0.0†	0.0†	0.0†
1–2	3.0	49.5	0.0†	0.0†	0.0†	49.5	.2†	7.9	31.4	26.2	4.0	19.5	17.9	1.8†
3–5	4.7	70.7	0.0†	0.0†	0.0†	70.7	.9†	8.2	40.4	38.3	2.8	36.1	32.2	4.0
5 and under	8.8	55.4	0.0†	0.0†	0.0†	55.4	.6†	7.1	33.1	29.8	3.2	25.9	23.2	2.7
Males:														
6–11	4.6	71.8	.5†	0.0†	0.0†	71.8	1.5†	7.4	36.1	32.9	3.9†	46.0	41.7	6.1
12–19	5.9	86.4	3.8†	0.0†	2.4†	85.9	5.4	16.6	32.1	23.0	9.1	67.2	64.5	4.3
20–29	7.2	90.3	24.9	2.5†	21.5	85.8	24.9	16.0	19.3	16.0	3.6	67.8	63.0	6.8
30–39	8.1	92.8	22.4	2.6†	18.2	91.1	49.2	24.9	14.2	10.8	3.4	63.2	52.8	13.0
40–49	7.0	95.0	26.0	7.5	15.8	92.7	63.0	25.1	18.5	14.9	3.8†	54.2	42.0	14.9
50–59	4.7	95.3	22.2	4.6	14.9	94.1	67.1	31.6	12.2	8.7	2.4†	51.1	34.8	18.2
60–69	3.4	97.5†	18.9	7.7	9.7	96.8†	74.7	30.0	9.2	8.4	.9†	38.5	24.6	15.3
70 and over	3.4	91.8	14.6	7.1	3.6†	89.7	77.1	23.8	11.3	9.6	2.7†	22.4	12.7	9.7
20 and over	33.9	93.5	22.5	4.8	15.6	91.2	54.8	24.4	15.1	12.1	3.1	54.1	43.3	12.7
Females:														
6–11	4.4	69.4	.5†	0.0†	0.0†	69.4	1.3†	7.7	32.2	30.3	1.9†	45.2	41.2	6.3
12–19	5.6	86.7	1.7†	.5†	1.1†	86.7	4.9	17.1	25.5	21.3	4.1†	62.8	58.0	5.9
20–29	6.9	88.9	10.7	1.2†	7.4	87.0	26.2	23.5	22.4	18.4	3.5†	64.3	52.9	14.1
30–39	8.6	88.5	14.0	4.0	7.0	87.9	43.9	27.6	19.9	18.0	1.9†	55.0	39.6	18.9
40–49	7.2	93.8	15.9	7.9	6.8	93.4	60.1	30.4	15.0	13.0	2.2†	57.0	35.1	24.3
50–59	5.1	92.9	11.5	5.1	2.5†	91.9	63.3	37.9	13.4	11.2	1.0†	44.2	28.7	18.9
60–69	3.9	95.8†	12.8	6.5	1.9†	94.4	74.9	31.9	12.1	9.2	2.9†	40.2	20.9	19.9
70 and over	5.1	87.5	5.7†	5.2†	.5†	87.5	71.6	21.8	13.7	12.3	1.4†	19.5	11.3	7.3
20 and over	36.8	90.9	12.1	4.8	5.0	90.0	53.6	28.5	16.8	14.5	2.2	49.2	33.8	17.6
All individuals	100.0	86.3	12.4	3.4	7.3	85.2	39.0	22.0	20.6	17.5	3.1	50.3	39.9	12.2

†Estimates based on small cell sizes may tend to be less statistically reliable than estimates based on larger cell sizes. Cell size refers to the unweighted number of individuals in a given sex-age group or demographic group.

Note: Excludes breast-fed children.

SOURCE: "Beverages: Percentages of individuals consuming foods from various food groups, by sex and age, 1 day, 1996" in *Results From USDA's 1996 Continuing Survey of Food Intakes by Individuals and 1996 Diet and Health Knowledge Survey,* U.S. Agricultural Research Service, Beltsville, MD, 1997

Sweeteners

Total per capita consumption of caloric sweeteners, mainly sucrose (table sugar made from cane and beets) and corn sweeteners (high-fructose corn syrup), increased 26 percent from 123.0 pounds in 1980 to 155.1 pounds in 1998. (See Table 2.8 and Figure 2.10.) This amounted to over two-fifths of a pound of caloric sweeteners per person per day.

COMPARISON OF PER CAPITA CONSUMPTION AND USDA RECOMMENDATIONS

A Dietary Assessment of the U.S. Food Supply: Comparing Per Capita Food Consumption with Food Guide Pyramid Serving Recommendations (Linda Scott Kantor, Economic Research Service, USDA, Washington, D.C., 1998), the first study of its kind, compared average diets with the federal dietary recommendations. It used data from the food supply series *Food Consumption, Prices, and Expenditures, 1970–95* (Judith Jones Putnam and Jane E. Allshouse, Economic Research Service, USDA, Washington, D.C., 1997). The study was based on a sample diet of 2,200 calories, a daily energy intake considered by the USDA as appropriate for most children, teenage girls, active women, and sedentary men.

Grain Group

The study found that, in 1996, the grains group (bread, cereals, rice, and pasta) was the only food group that met the total servings recommended by the Food Guide Pyramid. (See Table 2.9 and Figure 2.11.) On the other hand, although Americans are eating more grain products, these are mostly refined, rather than high-fiber, whole-grain products. In 1996, of the 148.7 pounds of wheat flour consumed per capita (Table 2.8), less than 2 percent was whole-wheat flour. This finding was confirmed by the 1996 *Continuing Survey of Food Intakes by Individuals* (CSFII), which found that the mean daily intake of foods made from whole grains constituted just one serving of the Food Guide Pyramid recommendation.

During the processing and refining of whole grains, the bran and germ (fiber) are removed, as well as such nutrients as vitamins and minerals. Even when the finished product has been "enriched" with some vitamins

TABLE 2.7

Percent of individuals consuming various types of eggs, legumes, nuts and seeds, fats and oils, and sugars and sweets over the course of one day, by sex and age, 1996

Sex and age (years)	Percentage of population	Eggs	Legumes	Nuts and seeds	Fats and oils			Sugars and sweets		
					Total	Table fats	Salad dressings	Total	Sugars	Candy
	Percent				Percent					
Males and females:										
Under 1	1.1	9.4†	19.7	1.8†	5.3†	5.3†	0.0†	9.5†	1.3†	0.0†
1–2	3.0	25.5	10.2	15.9	35.0	26.4	10.8	45.7	10.6	14.7
3–5	4.7	17.3	7.8	19.5	37.6	25.8	16.2	62.6	14.0	26.9
5 and under	8.8	19.1	10.2	16.0	32.5	23.3	12.3	50.0	11.2	19.3
Males:										
6–11	4.6	11.2	10.1	11.4	45.2	29.4	23.4	55.0	12.2	28.0
12–19	5.9	16.7	11.8	8.8	40.6	16.4	29.2	43.3	9.0	21.4
20–29	7.2	21.8	13.7	6.9	46.6	17.8	32.3	39.4	19.1	16.1
30–39	8.1	20.1	17.5	7.5	56.4	24.7	31.9	49.3	32.4	12.3
40–49	7.0	21.9	15.6	6.5	60.8	32.3	31.7	53.8	36.9	10.2
50–59	4.7	24.4	16.0	11.9	60.0	36.7	32.6	56.8	42.3	8.4
60–69	3.4	26.2	19.0	8.4	69.9	39.8	39.0	62.7	44.7	13.6
70 and over	3.4	27.6	16.3	12.0	68.0	48.3	34.7	62.1	41.3	7.0
20 and over	33.9	22.8	16.1	8.3	58.3	30.4	33.0	51.8	34.0	11.7
Females:										
6–11	4.4	11.0	12.5	17.7	44.3	28.9	18.8	63.3	11.0	26.7
12–19	5.6	11.6	9.6	7.1	49.3	24.4	33.1	45.2	11.1	26.7
20–29	6.9	18.1	18.6	5.4	48.9	29.2	26.3	43.9	26.1	11.3
30–39	8.6	16.2	16.9	8.6	59.8	29.6	32.3	55.6	36.9	13.3
40–49	7.2	21.1	16.4	5.7	63.6	34.1	38.7	52.2	36.0	13.9
50–59	5.1	16.0	16.1	6.2	66.9	33.5	40.1	66.5	45.0	13.5
60–69	3.9	26.3	15.3	8.6	65.0	37.9	37.0	55.9	38.9	7.9
70 and over	5.1	21.4	10.9	9.3	63.6	42.3	29.8	54.9	29.8	10.6
20 and over	36.8	19.3	16.0	7.2	60.6	33.6	33.7	54.2	35.1	12.1
All individuals	100.0	19.1	14.5	9.1	54.1	29.7	30.1	52.3	27.6	15.4

†Estimates based on small cell sizes may tend to be less statistically reliable than estimates based on larger cell sizes. Cell size refers to the unweighted number of individuals in a given sex-age group or demographic group.

Note: Excludes breast-fed children.

SOURCE: "Eggs; legumes; nuts and seeds; fats and oils; sugars and sweets: Percentages of individuals consuming foods from various food groups, by sex and age, 1 day, 1996" in *Results From USDA's 1996 Continuing Survey of Food Intakes by Individuals and 1996 Diet and Health Knowledge Survey,* U.S. Agricultural Research Service, Beltsville, MD, 1997

and minerals or fiber, many of the initial nutrients have been lost.

Whole-grain products always list whole wheat or another whole grain (oats, whole rye, brown and wild rice) as the first ingredient. Descriptions, such as "100 percent wheat," "multigrain," or "7-grain," may not necessarily mean the product is made from whole grains. Oatmeal bread, for example, may not necessarily be a whole-grain product unless oats are listed as the first ingredient.

Vegetable Group

In 1996 the daily per capita consumption of 3.8 servings of vegetables almost equaled the Food Guide Pyramid recommendation of 4 servings. (See Table 2.9 and Figure 2.12.) *The Food Guide Pyramid* bulletin (Center for Nutrition Policy and Promotion, USDA, Home and Garden Bulletin No. 252, 1996) further suggests dividing daily vegetable servings among deep yellow vegetables, dark green leafy vegetables, and starchy vegetables, including dry beans, peas, and lentils. Out of about 80 different vegetables considered by the ERS data, just 5 vegetables—head lettuce, 16.3 percent; frozen potatoes, 11.4 percent; fresh potatoes, 10 percent; potatoes for chips, 6.1 percent; and canned tomatoes, 5.9 percent—accounted for half of the total servings. (See Figure 2.13.)

Daily per capita consumption provided only one-tenth of a daily serving of dark green leafy vegetables (mostly from broccoli and Romaine lettuce) and less than one-quarter of a daily serving of deep yellow vegetables (more than 75 percent of which were from fresh, frozen, and canned carrots). Similarly, the 1996 CSFII data reported that survey participants satisfied just 6 percent of the Food Guide Pyramid recommendation for dark green leafy vegetables.

Fruit Group

The 1996 daily per capita consumption of fruits provided just 1.3 servings, not even half the Food Guide Pyramid recommendation of 3 servings. (See Table 2.9 and

FIGURE 2.1

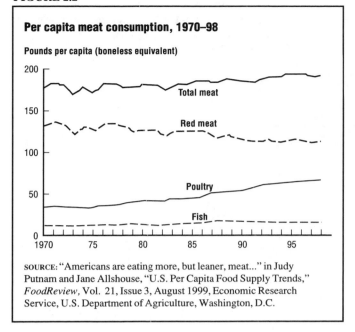

Estimating U.S. food consumption: the supply-and-utilization commodity flow

SOURCE: "Estimating U.S. Food Consumption: The Supply and Utilization Commodity Flow" in Judith Jones Putnam and Jane E. Allshouse, *Food Consumption, Prices, and Expenditures, 1970–95*, Economic Research Service, U.S. Department of Agriculture, Washington, D.C., 1997

FIGURE 2.3

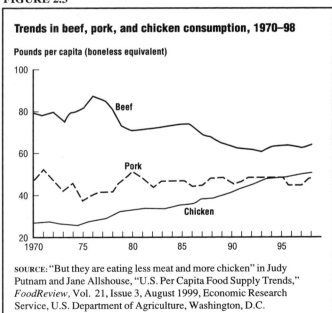

Trends in beef, pork, and chicken consumption, 1970–98

Pounds per capita (boneless equivalent)

SOURCE: "But they are eating less meat and more chicken" in Judy Putnam and Jane Allshouse, "U.S. Per Capita Food Supply Trends," *FoodReview,* Vol. 21, Issue 3, August 1999, Economic Research Service, U.S. Department of Agriculture, Washington, D.C.

FIGURE 2.2

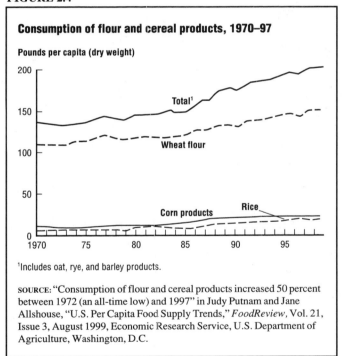

Per capita meat consumption, 1970–98

Pounds per capita (boneless equivalent)

SOURCE: "Americans are eating more, but leaner, meat..." in Judy Putnam and Jane Allshouse, "U.S. Per Capita Food Supply Trends," *FoodReview,* Vol. 21, Issue 3, August 1999, Economic Research Service, U.S. Department of Agriculture, Washington, D.C.

FIGURE 2.4

Consumption of flour and cereal products, 1970–97

Pounds per capita (dry weight)

[1]Includes oat, rye, and barley products.

SOURCE: "Consumption of flour and cereal products increased 50 percent between 1972 (an all-time low) and 1997" in Judy Putnam and Jane Allshouse, "U.S. Per Capita Food Supply Trends," *FoodReview,* Vol. 21, Issue 3, August 1999, Economic Research Service, U.S. Department of Agriculture, Washington, D.C.

Figure 2.14.) Moreover, consumers limited themselves to a few fruits, with half of the fruit servings coming from six fruits—orange juice, 18 percent; bananas, 9.8 percent; fresh apples, 7.9 percent; watermelon, 6.5 percent; apple juice, 5.8 percent; and fresh grapes, 5.1 percent.

Milk, Yogurt, and Cheese Group (Dairy Group)

The dairy group is the only food group whose recommendations are weighted based on age and physiological status rather than the total energy intake. Three servings are recommended for teenagers, young adults up to 24 years old, and pregnant and lactating women. For children and other adults, the Food Guide Pyramid recommendation is two daily servings from the dairy group.

TABLE 2.8

Per capita consumption of major food commodities, 1980–98

[In pounds, retail weight, except as indicated. Consumption represents the residual after exports, nonfood use and ending stocks are subtracted from the sum of beginning stocks, domestic production, and imports. Based on Census Bureau estimated population]

Commodity	Unit	1980	1985	1990	1995	1996	1997	1998
Red meat, total (boneless, trimmed weight) [1][2]	Pounds	126.4	124.9	112.3	115.1	112.8	111.0	115.6
Beef	Pounds	72.1	74.6	63.9	64.4	65.0	63.8	64.9
Veal	Pounds	1.3	1.5	0.9	0.8	1.0	0.9	0.7
Lamb and mutton	Pounds	1.0	1.1	1.0	0.9	0.8	0.8	0.9
Pork	Pounds	52.1	47.7	46.4	49.0	45.9	45.5	49.2
Poultry (boneless, trimmed weight) [2]	Pounds	40.8	45.5	56.3	62.9	64.1	64.2	65.0
Chicken	Pounds	32.7	36.4	42.4	48.8	49.5	50.4	50.8
Turkey	Pounds	8.1	9.1	13.8	14.1	14.6	13.9	14.2
Fish and shellfish (boneless, trimmed weight)	Pounds	12.4	15.0	15.0	14.9	14.7	14.5	14.8
Eggs	Number	271	255	234	235	237	239	244
Shell	Number	236	217	186	175	175	173	176
Processed	Number	35	38	48	61	62	66	58
Dairy products, total [3]	Pounds	543.2	593.7	568.4	583.9	574.7	577.7	582.3
Fluid milk products [4]	Gallons	27.9	27.1	26.2	24.9	24.9	24.6	24.3
Beverage milks	Gallons	27.6	26.7	25.7	24.3	24.4	24.0	23.7
Plain whole milk	Gallons	16.5	13.9	10.2	8.4	8.4	8.2	8.0
Plain reduced-fat milk (2%)	Gallons	6.3	7.9	9.1	8.2	8.0	7.7	7.5
Plain light and skim milks	Gallons	3.1	3.2	4.9	6.2	6.4	6.6	6.6
Flavored whole milk	Gallons	0.6	0.4	0.3	0.3	0.3	0.3	0.3
Flavored milks other than whole	Gallons	0.6	0.7	0.8	0.8	0.9	0.9	1.0
Buttermilk	Gallons	0.5	0.5	0.4	0.3	0.3	0.3	0.3
Yogurt (excl. frozen)	1/2 pints	4.6	7.3	7.4	9.4	8.9	9.5	9.3
Fluid cream products [5]	1/2 pints	10.5	13.5	14.3	15.9	16.4	17.0	17.3
Cream [6]	1/2 pints	6.3	8.2	8.7	9.5	10.2	10.7	10.9
Sour cream and dips	1/2 pints	3.4	4.3	4.7	5.5	5.4	5.6	5.7
Condensed and evaporated milks	Pounds	7.0	7.5	7.9	6.9	6.4	6.6	6.4
Whole milk	Pounds	3.8	3.6	3.2	2.3	2.3	2.6	2.2
Skim milk	Pounds	3.3	3.8	4.8	4.5	4.1	4.0	4.1
Cheese [7]	Pounds	17.5	22.5	24.6	27.3	27.7	28.0	28.4
American	Pounds	9.6	12.2	11.1	11.8	12.0	12.0	12.2
Cheddar	Pounds	6.9	9.8	9.0	9.1	9.2	9.6	9.6
Italian	Pounds	4.4	6.5	9.0	10.4	10.8	11.0	11.3
Mozzarella	Pounds	.0	4.6	6.9	8.1	8.5	8.4	8.7
Other [8]	Pounds	3.4	3.9	4.5	5.0	5.0	5.0	4.8
Swiss	Pounds	1.3	1.3	1.4	1.1	1.1	1.0	1.0
Cream and Neufchatel	Pounds	1.0	1.2	1.7	2.1	2.2	2.3	2.3
Cottage cheese, total	Pounds	4.5	4.1	3.4	2.7	2.6	2.7	2.7
Lowfat	Pounds	0.8	1.0	1.2	1.2	1.2	1.3	1.3
Frozen dairy products	Pounds	26.4	27.9	28.4	29.4	28.6	28.8	29.6
Ice cream	Pounds	17.5	18.1	15.8	15.7	15.9	16.4	16.6
Lowfat ice cream	Pounds	7.1	6.9	7.7	7.5	7.6	7.9	8.3
Sherbet	Pounds	1.2	1.3	1.2	1.3	1.3	1.3	1.4
Frozen yogurt	Pounds	(NA)	(NA)	2.8	3.5	2.6	2.1	1.9
Fats and oils:								
Total, fat content only	Pounds	56.9	64.1	63.0	66.4	65.3	64.9	65.3
Butter (product weight)	Pounds	4.5	4.9	4.4	4.5	4.3	4.2	4.2
Margarine (product weight)	Pounds	11.3	10.8	10.9	9.2	9.2	8.6	8.3
Lard (direct use)	Pounds	2.3	1.6	1.6	1.7	1.8	1.9	2.0
Edible beef tallow (direct use)	Pounds	1.1	2.0	0.6	2.7	3.0	2.2	3.2
Shortening	Pounds	18.2	22.9	22.2	22.5	22.3	20.9	20.9
Salad and cooking oils	Pounds	21.3	23.6	25.3	26.9	26.2	28.6	27.9
Other edible fats and oils	Pounds	1.5	1.6	1.2	1.6	1.4	1.1	1.3
Flour and cereal products [9]	Pounds	144.7	156.5	181.5	190.7	196.4	197.1	196.8
Wheat flour	Pounds	116.9	124.6	136.0	141.9	148.7	149.5	147.8
Rice, milled	Pounds	9.4	9.1	15.8	18.9	17.8	18.5	18.9
Corn products	Pounds	12.9	17.2	21.9	21.8	21.9	21.8	22.3
Oat products	Pounds	3.9	4.0	6.5	6.5	6.6	6.6	6.6
Breakfast cereals [10]	Pounds	12.0	12.8	15.4	17.1	16.9	16.9	(NA)
Ready-to-eat	Pounds	9.7	10.5	12.6	14.6	14.3	14.3	(NA)
Ready-to-cook	Pounds	2.3	2.3	2.9	2.5	2.5	2.6	(NA)
Caloric sweeteners, total [11]	Pounds	123.0	128.8	137.0	149.8	150.7	154.0	155.1
Sugar, refined cane and beet	Pounds	83.6	62.7	64.4	65.5	66.5	66.5	67.0
Corn sweeteners [12]	Pounds	38.2	64.8	71.1	83.0	82.8	86.2	86.8
High-fructose corn syrup	Pounds	19.0	45.2	49.6	58.4	59.4	62.5	63.8
Other:								
Cocoa beans	Pounds	3.4	4.6	5.4	4.6	5.3	5.1	(NA)
Coffee (green beans)	Pounds	10.3	10.5	10.3	8.0	8.9	9.3	9.5
Peanuts (shelled)	Pounds	4.8	6.3	6.0	5.7	5.7	5.9	5.9
Tree nuts (shelled)	Pounds	1.8	2.5	2.5	2.4	1.9	2.0	2.3

NA Not available. [1] Excludes edible offals. [2] Excludes shipments to Puerto Rico and the other U.S possessions. [3] Milk-equivalent, milkfat basis. Includes butter. [4] Fluid milk figures are aggregates of commercial sales and milk produced and consumed on farms. [5] Includes eggnog, not shown separately. [6] Heavy cream, light cream, and half and half. [7] Excludes full-skim American, cottage, pot, and bakers cheese. [8] Includes other cheeses not shown separately. [9] Includes rye flour and barley products not shown separately. Excludes quantities used in alcoholic beverages. [10] Partially overlaps flour and cereal products category. [11] Dry weight. Includes edible syrups (maple, molasses, etc.) and honey not shown separately. [12] Includes glucose and dextrose not shown separately.

SOURCE: "Per Capita Consumption of Major Food Commodities: 1980 to 1998" in *Statistical Abstract of the United States, 2000*, U.S. Census Bureau, Washington, D.C., 2000

Nutrition: A Key to Good Health

FIGURE 2.5

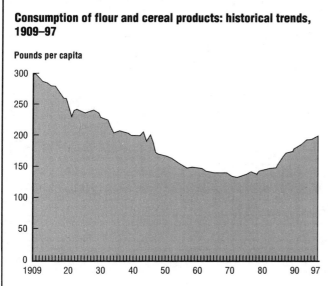

Consumption of flour and cereal products: historical trends, 1909–97

Pounds per capita

SOURCE: "But in 1997, it remained 100 pounds below the 1909 level" in Judy Putnam and Jane Allshouse, "U.S. Per Capita Food Supply Trends," *FoodReview*, Vol. 21, Issue 3, August 1999, Economic Research Service, U.S. Department of Agriculture, Washington, D.C.

FIGURE 2.6

Per capita consumption of fruits and vegetables: 1970, 1982, and 1997

Pounds per capita

[1]Publication of *Diet, Nutrition, and Cancer,* which emphasized the importance of fruit and vegetables in the daily diet.

SOURCE: "Fruit and vegetable consumption increased 19 percent from 1982 to 1997" in Judy Putnam and Jane Allshouse, "U.S. Per Capita Food Supply Trends," *FoodReview*, Vol. 21, Issue 3, August 1999, Economic Research Service, U.S. Department of Agriculture, Washington, D.C.

FIGURE 2.7

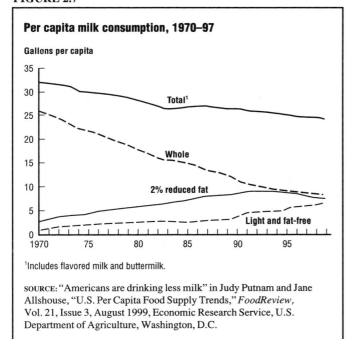

Per capita milk consumption, 1970–97

Gallons per capita

[1]Includes flavored milk and buttermilk.

SOURCE: "Americans are drinking less milk" in Judy Putnam and Jane Allshouse, "U.S. Per Capita Food Supply Trends," *FoodReview*, Vol. 21, Issue 3, August 1999, Economic Research Service, U.S. Department of Agriculture, Washington, D.C.

FIGURE 2.8

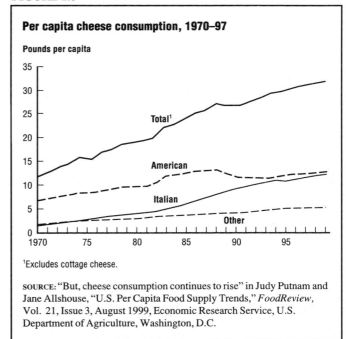

Per capita cheese consumption, 1970–97

Pounds per capita

[1]Excludes cottage cheese.

SOURCE: "But, cheese consumption continues to rise" in Judy Putnam and Jane Allshouse, "U.S. Per Capita Food Supply Trends," *FoodReview*, Vol. 21, Issue 3, August 1999, Economic Research Service, U.S. Department of Agriculture, Washington, D.C.

In 1996 the daily per capita consumption provided 1.7 servings of dairy products, somewhat short of the Pyramid recommendation of 2.2 servings daily. (See Table 2.9 and Figure 2.15.) More than half of the dairy products consumed came from natural and processed cheese (38 percent) and whole milk (16 percent), which included dry and condensed milk. One-quarter of the servings were provided by skim milk (16 percent); low fat, or 1 percent milk (5 percent); and yogurt and buttermilk (2 percent, most of which were low fat). Reduced-fat, or 2 percent milk, made up 15 percent of the servings, and ice cream and other frozen dairy desserts accounted for 4 percent of the total servings.

Dairy foods are typically high in fat content. USDA experts, in light of the steep rise in cheese consumption since 1970 (Figure 2.8), surmise that consumers are probably substituting one high-fat dairy food (cheese) for another (whole milk). They caution those who wish to increase their servings of dairy products to watch their total fat intake, since regular cheese generally has a higher proportion of total and saturated fat than whole milk.

Meat Group

In 1996 the daily per capita consumption (5.6 ounces, cooked) of foods in the meat group—red meat, poultry, fish, dry beans, eggs, and nuts—nearly equaled the Food Guide

Pyramid's recommended 6 ounces. The red-meat share (52 percent) of the total meat servings was nearly twice that of poultry (29 percent). Fish and shellfish made up 7 percent, and eggs accounted for 9 percent of the meat-group servings. Peanut butter comprised another 2 percent of the recommended servings. (See Table 2.9 and Figure 2.16.)

Although dry beans, peas, and lentils belong to the vegetable group, they are also included in the meat group

FIGURE 2.9

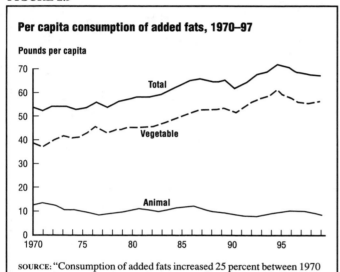

Per capita consumption of added fats, 1970–97

Pounds per capita

SOURCE: "Consumption of added fats increased 25 percent between 1970 and 1997" in Judy Putnam and Jane Allshouse, "U.S. Per Capita Food Supply Trends," *FoodReview*, Vol. 21, Issue 3, August 1999, Economic Research Service, U.S. Department of Agriculture, Washington, D.C.

FIGURE 2.10

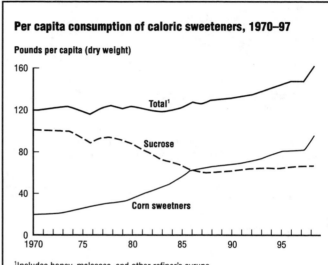

Per capita consumption of caloric sweeteners, 1970–97

Pounds per capita (dry weight)

[1]Includes honey, malasses, and other refiner's syrups.

SOURCE: "Caloric sweetener consumption rose 26 percent from 1970 to 1997; 85 percent of that increase occurred since 1986" in Judy Putnam and Jane Allshouse, "U.S. Per Capita Food Supply Trends," *FoodReview*, Vol. 21, Issue 3, August 1999, Economic Research Service, U.S. Department of Agriculture, Washington, D.C.

TABLE 2.9

Average food supply servings for 1970–96 compared with Food Guide Pyramid serving recommendations

Food group	Servings				Food Guide Pyramid serving recommendation[1]
	1970–75	1980–85	1990–95	1996	
Grains	6.8	7.5	9.2	9.7	9
Vegetables	3.1	3.2	3.6	3.8	4
Fruits	1.1	1.2	1.3	1.3	3
Milk, yogurt, and cheese[2]	1.6	1.5	1.6	1.7	2.2
Meat, poultry, fish, dry beans, eggs, and nuts (ounces)	5.4	5.5	5.6	5.6	6.0
Added fats and oils (grams of fat)[3]	49	55	62	60	38
Added sugars (teaspoons)[4]	27	26	31	32	12

[1] Recommendation based on a 2,200-calorie diet. A 2,200-calorie diet is close to the 2,247 calories recommended as an average caloric intake for the population in 1995. Recommended servings for other years may differ.

[2] Three servings of milk, yogurt, and cheese are appropriate for teenagers and young adults to age 24 and for pregnant and breastfeeding women. Two servings are recommended for other adults.

[3] *The 1996 Dietary Guidelines* recommend that consumers choose a diet that provides no more than 30 percent of total calories from fat. The upper limit on the grams of fat in a consumer's diet will depend on calorie intake. For example, for a person consuming 2,200 calories per day, the upper limit on total daily fat intake is 660 calories. Seventy-three grams of fat contribute about 660 calories (73 grams x 9 calories per gram of fat = 660 calories). According to food supply data for 1994, added fats and oils account for 52 percent of the total fat provided by the food supply in that year. The recommendation shown here assumes that added fats and oils account for 52 percent of total fat intake for a daily upper limit of 38 grams of added fats and oils (73 * 0.52) = 38.

[4] To avoid getting too many calories from sugar, dietary guidance suggests that consumers on a 2,200-calorie diet try to limit added sugars to the daily quantity listed.

SOURCE: Linda Scott Kantor, *A Dietary Assessment of the U.S. Food Supply: Comparing Per Capita Food Consumption with Food Guide Serving Recommendations,* U.S. Department of Agriculture, Economic Research Service, Washington, D.C., 1998

FIGURE 2.11

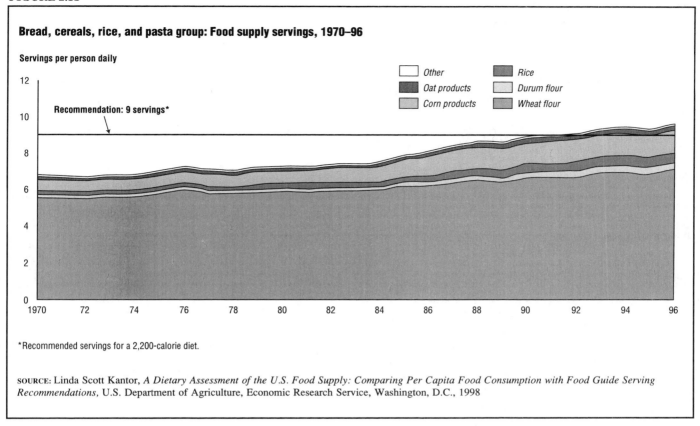

Bread, cereals, rice, and pasta group: Food supply servings, 1970–96

Servings per person daily

Legend:
- Other
- Oat products
- Corn products
- Rice
- Durum flour
- Wheat flour

Recommendation: 9 servings*

*Recommended servings for a 2,200-calorie diet.

SOURCE: Linda Scott Kantor, *A Dietary Assessment of the U.S. Food Supply: Comparing Per Capita Food Consumption with Food Guide Serving Recommendations,* U.S. Department of Agriculture, Economic Research Service, Washington, D.C., 1998

FIGURE 2.12

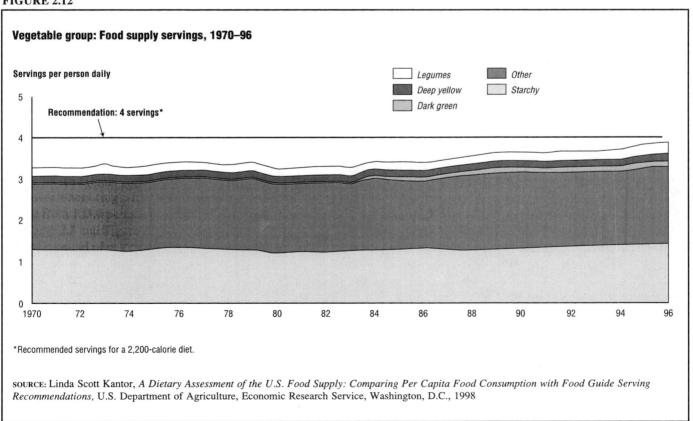

Vegetable group: Food supply servings, 1970–96

Servings per person daily

Legend:
- Legumes
- Deep yellow
- Dark green
- Other
- Starchy

Recommendation: 4 servings*

*Recommended servings for a 2,200-calorie diet.

SOURCE: Linda Scott Kantor, *A Dietary Assessment of the U.S. Food Supply: Comparing Per Capita Food Consumption with Food Guide Serving Recommendations,* U.S. Department of Agriculture, Economic Research Service, Washington, D.C., 1998

FIGURE 2.13

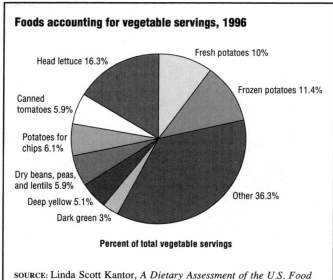

Foods accounting for vegetable servings, 1996

Head lettuce 16.3%
Fresh potatoes 10%
Frozen potatoes 11.4%
Canned tomatoes 5.9%
Potatoes for chips 6.1%
Dry beans, peas, and lentils 5.9%
Deep yellow 5.1%
Dark green 3%
Other 36.3%

Percent of total vegetable servings

SOURCE: Linda Scott Kantor, *A Dietary Assessment of the U.S. Food Supply: Comparing Per Capita Food Consumption with Food Guide Serving Recommendations,* U.S. Department of Agriculture, Economic Research Service, Washington, D.C., 1998

because they are an excellent source of protein. They are low in fat, high in fiber, and cost less than meat, poultry, or fish.

Added Fats and Oils

In 1996 the typical American consumed 60 grams of overall added fats and oils a day. Since the 1980s salad and cooking oils and shortening have accounted for more than two-thirds of the total added fat and oil servings in the diet and for almost all the increase in added fat and oil use. (See Figure 2.17 and Table 2.10.)

Added Sugars

In 1996 the daily per capita consumption of added sugars was 32 teaspoons of caloric sweeteners. Caloric sweetener consumption rose 26 percent from 1970 to 1997, with 85 percent of that increase occurring since 1986. (See Figure 2.8.) Part of that increase is due to the consumption of nondiet carbonated soft drinks, which increased 47 percent from 1986 to 1997. (See Figure 2.18.) According to the *Food Guide Pyramid* bulletin, persons on a 1,600-calorie diet should limit their added sugar intake to 6 teaspoons per day. The suggested upper limit for a 2,200-calorie diet is 12 teaspoons and for a 2,800-calorie diet, 18 teaspoons of added sugar.

FIGURE 2.14

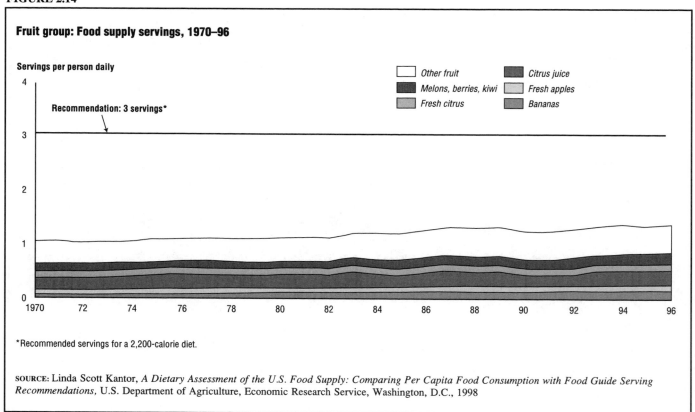

Fruit group: Food supply servings, 1970–96

Servings per person daily

Recommendation: 3 servings*

Other fruit
Melons, berries, kiwi
Fresh citrus
Citrus juice
Fresh apples
Bananas

*Recommended servings for a 2,200-calorie diet.

SOURCE: Linda Scott Kantor, *A Dietary Assessment of the U.S. Food Supply: Comparing Per Capita Food Consumption with Food Guide Serving Recommendations,* U.S. Department of Agriculture, Economic Research Service, Washington, D.C., 1998

FIGURE 2.15

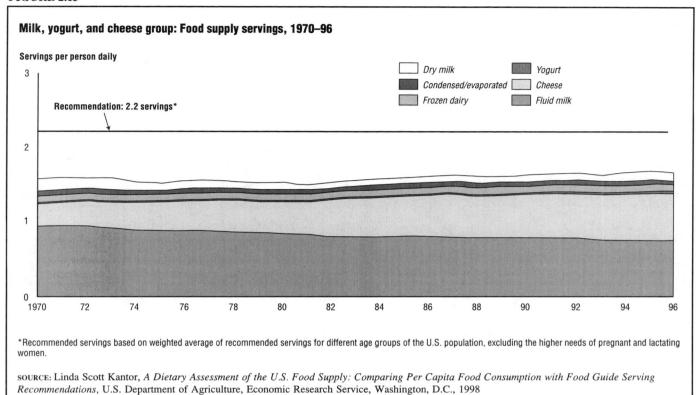

Milk, yogurt, and cheese group: Food supply servings, 1970–96

Servings per person daily

Legend: Dry milk, Condensed/evaporated, Frozen dairy, Yogurt, Cheese, Fluid milk

Recommendation: 2.2 servings*

*Recommended servings based on weighted average of recommended servings for different age groups of the U.S. population, excluding the higher needs of pregnant and lactating women.

SOURCE: Linda Scott Kantor, *A Dietary Assessment of the U.S. Food Supply: Comparing Per Capita Food Consumption with Food Guide Serving Recommendations,* U.S. Department of Agriculture, Economic Research Service, Washington, D.C., 1998

FIGURE 2.16

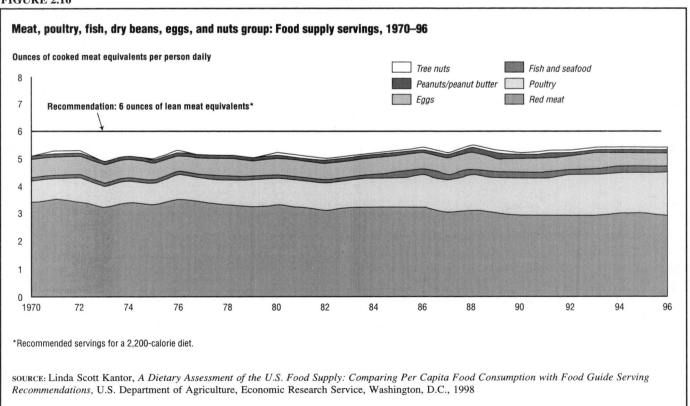

Meat, poultry, fish, dry beans, eggs, and nuts group: Food supply servings, 1970–96

Ounces of cooked meat equivalents per person daily

Legend: Tree nuts, Peanuts/peanut butter, Eggs, Fish and seafood, Poultry, Red meat

Recommendation: 6 ounces of lean meat equivalents*

*Recommended servings for a 2,200-calorie diet.

SOURCE: Linda Scott Kantor, *A Dietary Assessment of the U.S. Food Supply: Comparing Per Capita Food Consumption with Food Guide Serving Recommendations,* U.S. Department of Agriculture, Economic Research Service, Washington, D.C., 1998

FIGURE 2.17

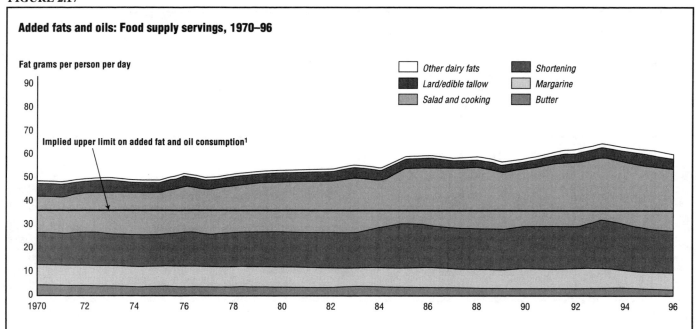

Added fats and oils: Food supply servings, 1970–96

Fat grams per person per day

Legend:
- Other dairy fats
- Lard/edible tallow
- Salad and cooking
- Shortening
- Margarine
- Butter

Implied upper limit on added fat and oil consumption[1]

[1]Implied upper limit assumes 2,200-calorie diet and that added fats account for 52 percent of suggested upper limit on total fat intake of 73 grams or 30 percent of calories.

SOURCE: Linda Scott Kantor, *A Dietary Assessment of the U.S. Food Supply: Comparing Per Capita Food Consumption with Food Guide Serving Recommendations,* U.S. Department of Agriculture, Economic Research Service, Washington, D.C., 1998

FIGURE 2.18

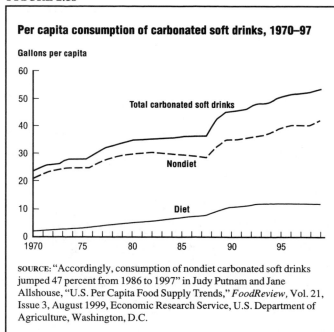

Per capita consumption of carbonated soft drinks, 1970–97

Gallons per capita

Total carbonated soft drinks

Nondiet

Diet

SOURCE: "Accordingly, consumption of nondiet carbonated soft drinks jumped 47 percent from 1986 to 1997" in Judy Putnam and Jane Allshouse, "U.S. Per Capita Food Supply Trends," *FoodReview,* Vol. 21, Issue 3, August 1999, Economic Research Service, U.S. Department of Agriculture, Washington, D.C.

TABLE 2.10

Per capita consumption of added fats and oils, 1960–97

| Year | Table spreads | | | Baking and frying fats | | | Salad, cooking, and other edible oils | Total |
	Butter	Margarine	Total	Lard and tallow[1]	Shortening	Total		
				Pounds				
1960	6.1	7.5	13.6	7.5	12.6	20.1	11.5	45.2
1961	6.0	7.5	13.5	7.6	12.9	20.4	11.2	45.1
1962	6.0	7.3	13.4	7.1	13.4	20.5	11.7	45.6
1963	5.7	7.6	13.2	6.3	13.5	19.8	13.2	46.3
1964	5.7	7.7	13.3	6.2	13.8	20.0	14.2	47.5
1965	5.3	7.8	13.2	6.3	14.2	20.5	14.1	47.7
1966	4.6	8.5	13.1	5.5	16.0	21.4	15.1	49.6
1967	4.4	8.4	12.8	5.3	15.9	21.3	15.1	49.2
1968	4.7	8.5	13.2	5.5	16.3	21.8	15.9	50.9
1969	4.5	8.6	13.1	5.0	17.0	22.0	16.5	51.6
1970	4.3	8.7	13.0	4.6	17.3	21.9	17.7	52.6
1971	4.1	8.7	12.9	4.2	16.8	21.0	17.9	51.8
1972	4.0	8.9	12.9	3.7	17.6	21.4	19.1	53.4
1973	3.8	8.9	12.7	3.3	17.0	20.4	20.3	53.3
1974	3.6	8.9	12.5	3.2	16.9	20.1	19.8	52.4
1975	3.8	8.8	12.6	3.2	17.0	20.2	19.9	52.6
1976	3.5	9.5	13.0	2.9	17.7	20.6	21.5	55.1
1977	3.4	9.1	12.5	2.5	17.2	19.8	21.0	53.3
1978	3.5	9.0	12.5	2.4	17.8	20.2	22.2	54.9
1979	3.6	8.9	12.5	2.9	18.4	21.3	22.5	56.4
1980	3.6	9.0	12.6	3.6	18.2	21.8	22.7	57.2
1981	3.4	8.9	12.3	3.5	18.5	21.9	23.2	57.4
1982	3.5	8.8	12.3	3.8	18.6	22.4	23.5	58.3
1983	3.9	8.3	12.2	4.1	18.5	22.6	25.1	60.0
1984	3.9	8.3	12.2	3.8	21.3	25.0	24.2	61.5
1985	3.9	8.6	12.5	3.7	22.9	26.6	25.2	64.3
1986	3.7	9.1	12.8	3.5	22.1	25.6	26.1	64.5
1987	3.7	8.4	12.1	2.7	21.4	24.1	26.9	63.1
1988	3.6	8.3	11.8	2.6	21.5	24.1	27.6	63.5
1989	3.5	8.1	11.6	2.1	21.5	23.5	25.7	60.8
1990	3.5	8.7	12.2	2.4	22.2	24.7	26.0	62.8
1991	3.5	8.5	11.9	3.1	22.4	25.5	28.0	65.4
1992	3.5	8.8	12.3	4.1	22.4	26.5	28.6	67.4
1993	3.7	8.9	12.6	3.9	25.1	29.0	28.5	70.2
1994	3.9	7.9	11.8	4.7	24.1	28.9	27.9	68.6
1995	3.6	7.4	11.0	4.9	22.5	27.4	28.5	66.9
1996	3.5	7.3	10.8	5.3	22.3	27.5	27.5	65.8
1997	3.3	6.9	10.2	4.7	20.9	25.6	29.8	65.6

[1]Direct use; excludes use in margarine and shortening.

SOURCE: "U.S. Per Capita Consumption of Added Fats and Oils" in Scott Sanford and Jane Allshouse, "Have We Turned the Corner on Fat Consumption?" *FoodReview,* Vol. 21, Issue 3, August 1999, Economic Research Service, U.S. Department of Agriculture, Washington, D.C.

CHAPTER 3
THE ROLE OF FOODS

Unless care is exercised in selecting food, a diet may result which is one-sided or badly balanced—that is, one in which either protein or fuel ingredients (carbohydrate and fat) are provided in excess . . . . The evils of overeating may not be felt at once, but sooner or later they are sure to appear—perhaps in an excessive amount of fatty tissue, perhaps in general debility, perhaps in actual disease.

— 1902; W. O. Atwater, first director of the Office of Experiment Stations in the USDA and author of the first USDA dietary guide, the *Farmers' Bulletin* of 1894

For centuries people have understood that there is a connection between the food they eat and their health, but diets have been generally limited to locally available foods and, for the poor, foods they could grow or catch. It is only in modern times and in developed countries that a broad range of foods has been available, giving people the option of eating a diversified, healthy diet.

As recently as a generation ago, good nutrition primarily meant preventing vitamin and mineral deficiencies and the diseases that stemmed from them. Today consumers expect more; they hope that their diets will help them remain active, live longer, and avoid illness. As more research has been done, our understanding of nutrition has had to change. What may have been considered solid scientific knowledge 10 years ago is questioned today, and what we accept today may well be wrong tomorrow. Nonetheless, nutritionists in the United States generally agree on what to eat and not eat to promote health and avoid disorders such as coronary heart disease, cancer, hypertension, and obesity.

DIETARY GUIDELINES FOR AMERICANS

Nutrition and Your Health: Dietary Guidelines for Americans, popularly referred to as *Dietary Guidelines,* was initially released jointly by the U.S. Department of Agriculture (USDA) and the U.S. Department of Health

TABLE 3.1

Dietary guidelines for Americans

• Aim for a healthy weight.
• Be physically active each day.

• Let the Pyramid guide your food choices.
• Choose a variety of grains daily, especially whole grains.
• Choose a variety of fruits and vegetables daily.
• Keep food safe to eat.

• Choose a diet that is low in saturated fat and cholesterol and moderate in total fat.
• Choose beverages and foods to moderate your intake of sugars.
• Choose and prepare foods with less salt.
• If you drink alcoholic beverages, do so in moderation.

SOURCE: "Dietary Guidelines for Americans" in *Nutrition and Your Health: Dietary Guidelines for Americans,* U.S. Department of Agriculture, Washington, D.C., May 2000

and Human Services (HHS) in 1980. Under the National Nutrition Monitoring and Related Research Act of 1990 (PL 101-445), Congress mandated that the *Dietary Guidelines* be reviewed and revised, as needed, every five years. The act also required that every federal agency promote these guidelines.

The latest *Dietary Guidelines* was issued in 2000. Based on current scientific knowledge, the guidelines "are designed to help Americans choose diets that will meet nutrient requirements, promote health, support active lives, and reduce chronic disease risks." Table 3.1 presents the basic recommendations.

The Dietary Guidelines 2000 Advisory Committee was formed to revise the 1995 edition as mandated by Public Law 101-445. At its March 1999 meeting, the committee spoke of possible changes to the guidelines—focusing on "adequacy" of foods instead of "variety" and introducing different versions of the Food Guide Pyramid, such as Asian and Mediterranean versions. Other possible

FIGURE 3.1

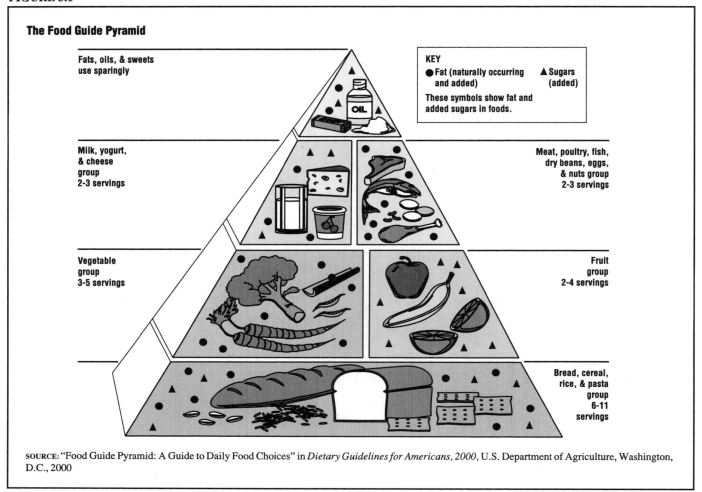

The Food Guide Pyramid

Fats, oils, & sweets use sparingly

KEY
● Fat (naturally occurring and added) ▲ Sugars (added)
These symbols show fat and added sugars in foods.

Milk, yogurt, & cheese group
2-3 servings

Meat, poultry, fish, dry beans, eggs, & nuts group
2-3 servings

Vegetable group
3-5 servings

Fruit group
2-4 servings

Bread, cereal, rice, & pasta group
6-11 servings

SOURCE: "Food Guide Pyramid: A Guide to Daily Food Choices" in *Dietary Guidelines for Americans, 2000,* U.S. Department of Agriculture, Washington, D.C., 2000

changes included identifying the benefits of mono- and polyunsaturated fats and creating two guidelines for plant foods, one for grains and another for fruits and vegetables.

THE FOOD GUIDE PYRAMID

Two other federal guidelines—the Food Guide Pyramid and the Nutrition Guide Label—serve as educational tools to help consumers put the *Dietary Guidelines* into practice. The Food Guide Pyramid graphic (Figure 3.1) is published as part of a larger bulletin of dietary guidance, *The Food Guide Pyramid* bulletin, which explains the graphic's recommendations comprehensively.

The Food Guide Pyramid is not a rigid prescription, but a general guide to help consumers implement the *Dietary Guidelines* by suggesting both the types of food needed and the number of servings. The servings are only a general guide; there is no need for exact measurements. (See Table 3.2.) Nonetheless, if a person eats a significantly larger portion of food, he or she should count it as more than a serving. Table 3.3 shows how many servings of each food group are needed for several daily calorie intakes. If a person's calorie consump-

tion falls between categories, the number of servings can be estimated.

The Pyramid emphasizes foods from the bread, cereal, rice, and pasta group (6 to 11 servings) and the vegetable (3 to 5 servings) and fruit (2 to 4 servings) groups. Consumers are advised to choose more of their foods from the bread group at the base of the Pyramid. In addition, most people need to eat more fruit and vegetable servings in order to increase their intake of fiber, vitamins, and minerals.

Americans need only moderate amounts—2 to 3 servings each—from the milk group and the meat and beans group. Most foods in these groups come from animal sources.

The small tip of the Pyramid represents those foods that should be eaten sparingly. The fats, oils, and sweets group supplies calories but little or no vitamins and minerals.

FOOD GUIDE PYRAMID FOR YOUNG CHILDREN

In March 1999 the USDA introduced the *Food Guide Pyramid for Young Children,* targeted toward children ages

TABLE 3.2

What counts as a serving?

Bread, cereal, rice, and pasta group (grains group)—whole grain and refined
- 1 slice of bread
- About 1 cup of ready-to-eat cereal
- 1/2 cup of cooked cereal, rice, or pasta

Vegetable group
- 1 cup of raw leafy vegetables
- 1/2 cup of other vegetables—cooked or raw
- 3/4 cup of vegetable juice

Fruit group
- 1 medium apple, banana, orange, pear
- 1/2 cup of chopped, cooked, or canned fruit
- 3/4 cup of fruit juice

Milk, yogurt, and cheese group (milk group)*
- 1 cup of milk** or yogurt**
- 1 1/2 ounces of natural cheese** (such as Cheddar)
- 2 ounces of processed cheese** (such as American)

Meat, poultry, fish, dry beans, eggs, and nuts group (meat and beans group)
- 2–3 ounces of cooked lean meat, poultry, or fish
- 1/2 cup of cooked dry beans# or 1/2 cup of tofu counts as 1 ounce of lean meat
- 2 1/2-ounce soyburger or 1 egg counts as 1 ounce of lean meat
- 2 tablespoons of peanut butter or 1/3 cup of nuts counts as 1 ounce of lean meat

Note: Many of the serving sizes given above are smaller than those on the nutrition facts label. For example, 1 serving of cooked cereal, rice, or pasta is 1 cup for the label but only 1/2 cup for the Pyramid.

*This includes lactose-free and lactose-reduced milk products. One cup of soy-based beverage with added calcium is an option for those who prefer a non-dairy source of calcium.

**Choose fat-free or reduced-fat dairy products most often.

Dry beans, peas, and lentils can be counted as servings in either the meat and beans group or the vegetable group. As a vegetable, 1/2 cup of cooked, dry beans counts as 1 serving. As a meat substitute, 1 cup of cooked, dry beans counts as 1 serving (2 ounces of meat).

SOURCE: "What Counts as a Serving?" in *Dietary Guidelines for Americans, 2000*, U.S. Department of Agriculture, Washington, D.C., 2000

TABLE 3.3

Daily sample diets, by calorie level

	Lower about 1,600	Moderate about 2,200	Higher about 2,800
Grain group servings	6	8	11
Vegetable group servings	3	4	5
Fruit group serving	2	3	4
Milk group servings	2-3[1]	2-3[1]	2-3[1]
Meat group[2] (ounces)	5	6	7
Total fat (grams)	53	73	93
Total added sugars (teaspoons)	6	12	18

[1]Women who are pregnant or breastfeeding, teenagers, and young adults to age 24 need 3 servings.
[2]Meat group amounts are in total ounces.

SOURCE: "Sample Diets for a Day at 3 Calorie Levels" in *Food Guide Pyramid Booklet 2000*, Center for Nutrition Policy and Promotion, U.S. Department of Agriculture, Washington, D.C., 2000

two to six. (See Figure 3.2.) The new daily food guide is an offshoot of the original Pyramid, with emphasis on balanced meals, moderation, and variety in food choices, especially from the grain, fruit, and vegetable groups.

The Pyramid is based on the eating patterns of young children. Not surprisingly, two- to six-year-olds eat somewhat differently from older children and adults. More of their servings from the meat group come from ground beef and luncheon meat and less from fish. They are more likely to drink fruit juices than to eat whole fruits. They are less likely to eat lettuce salads and more likely to eat green beans. Young children are also more likely to consume ready-to-eat cereals.

The Pyramid has been simplified by shortening the name of food groups. Single numbers, instead of ranges, are used for servings. In addition, the graphic illustrates food items in single servings, when possible. The table at the bottom of the Pyramid shows what constitutes a single serving, (Figure 3.2) picturing the types of food most often eaten by children. Moreover, to encourage children to be physically active, the Pyramid features children playing.

Since some fats are needed for early growth and development, the *Food Guide Pyramid for Young Children* bul-

letin does not stress fat restrictions. Rather, it advises gradually changing from whole milk to lower-fat dairy products such as 2 percent or 1 percent or fat-free milk by age five. It also suggests eating lower-fat and lean meats instead of higher-fat varieties. The *Dietary Guidelines for Americans* suggests that, by age five, fat in preschoolers' diets be gradually reduced from the children's earlier levels (34 percent of total calories) to the level recommended for most people (no more than 30 percent of total calories).

DIET AND ILLNESS

Poor diets have long been known as a contributor to poor health. Table 3.4 outlines some consequences of over- and underconsumption of various nutrients. Poor diet has also been linked to several of the leading causes of death in the United States—diseases of the heart (coronary heart disease [CHD] and stroke) and malignant neoplasms (cancer). Diet also plays a major role in the development of diabetes, the sixth (women) and seventh (men) leading cause of death, as well as hypertension and overweight. In 1994 coronary heart disease, cancer, stroke, and diabetes cost society an estimated $70.9 billion in diet-related medical costs, lost productivity due to disability, and premature deaths (although factors suggest that this is a low estimate). Studies have shown that improved dietary habits could reduce deaths from CHD and stroke by at least 20 percent and cancer and diabetes mortality by at least 30 percent.

In "High Costs of Poor Eating Patterns in the United States" (*America's Eating Habits: Changes and Consequences*, USDA, Washington, D.C., 1999), Elizabeth Frazão notes that improving Americans' dietary habits would decrease morbidity and mortality associated with chronic health conditions. According to Frazão, in the United States, 14 percent of all deaths can be attributed to poor diets and/or sedentary lifestyles.

FIGURE 3.2

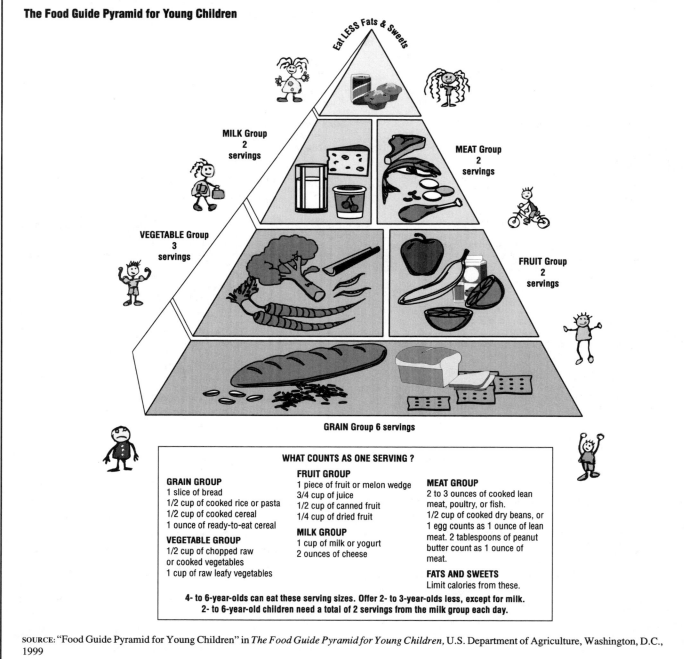

The Food Guide Pyramid for Young Children

Eat LESS Fats & Sweets

MILK Group
2
servings

MEAT Group
2
servings

VEGETABLE Group
3
servings

FRUIT Group
2
servings

GRAIN Group 6 servings

WHAT COUNTS AS ONE SERVING ?

GRAIN GROUP
1 slice of bread
1/2 cup of cooked rice or pasta
1/2 cup of cooked cereal
1 ounce of ready-to-eat cereal

VEGETABLE GROUP
1/2 cup of chopped raw
or cooked vegetables
1 cup of raw leafy vegetables

FRUIT GROUP
1 piece of fruit or melon wedge
3/4 cup of juice
1/2 cup of canned fruit
1/4 cup of dried fruit

MILK GROUP
1 cup of milk or yogurt
2 ounces of cheese

MEAT GROUP
2 to 3 ounces of cooked lean
meat, poultry, or fish.
1/2 cup of cooked dry beans, or
1 egg counts as 1 ounce of lean
meat. 2 tablespoons of peanut
butter count as 1 ounce of
meat.

FATS AND SWEETS
Limit calories from these.

**4- to 6-year-olds can eat these serving sizes. Offer 2- to 3-year-olds less, except for milk.
2- to 6-year-old children need a total of 2 servings from the milk group each day.**

SOURCE: "Food Guide Pyramid for Young Children" in *The Food Guide Pyramid for Young Children,* U.S. Department of Agriculture, Washington, D.C., 1999

DIETARY REFERENCE INTAKES (DRIS)

In the past, the Recommended Dietary Allowances (RDAs), prepared by the Food and Nutrition Board of the National Research Council under the National Academy of Sciences (NAS), served as the only standard of nutritional adequacy in the United States. Established in 1941, the RDAs are revised about every five years to reflect current scientific knowledge.

Due to the growing amount of scientific knowledge concerning the roles of nutrients, the NAS's Institute of Medicine, in partnership with the Canadian government, has revised the nutrient reference intakes. The new revised recommendations, called Dietary Reference Intakes (DRIs), include four reference values:

• Estimated Average Requirement (EAR)—the intake that meets the estimated nutrient need of half the individuals in a specific group. This figure is used as the basis for developing the new RDAs for some nutrients.

• Recommended Dietary Allowance (RDA)—the intake of essential nutrients that meets the known nutrient

TABLE 3.4

Consequence of inadequate and excessive intake of selected nutrients

Nutrient	Function in body	Consequence of inadequate intake	Consequence of excessive intake
Food energy	Metabolic processes; supports physical activity and growth, repairs bones and tissues, and maintains body temperature.	Underweight, semi-starvation, growth retardation in children.	Overweight and obesity (risk factors for heart disease, stroke, diabetes, hypertension, cancers).
Fiber	Promotes normal laxation.	Constipation; may increase risk of heart disease and some cancers.	Possible decrease in mineral absorption.
Calcium	Formation and maintenance of bone and teeth; muscle contraction; blood clotting; integrity of cell membranes.	May increase risk of osteoporosis.	Renal calculi; possible soft tissue calcification.
Iron	Carrier of oxygen in body; red blood cell formation.	Iron deficiency and iron deficiency anemia; functional impairments in intellectual development and learning, behavior, work performance, and resistance to infection.	Iron overload; may increase risk of stroke and some cancers in men.
Total fat, saturated fat, cholesterol	Concentrated sources of energy; carrier for fat-soluble vitamins; structural and functional components of cell membranes; precursors of compounds involved in many aspects of metabolism.	No public health problem; clinical deficiencies of essential fatty acids and fat-soluble nutrients have occurred.	Associated with elevated levels of blood cholesterol and of low-density lipoprotein (LDL) cholesterol, major risk factors for coronary heart disease.
Sodium	Regulation of body fluid volume and acid-base balance of blood; transmission of nerve impulses.	—	Edema; associated with high incidence of hypertension (risk factor for stroke and heart disease).

SOURCE: Lin, Biing-Hwan, Fazio, Elizabeth and Guthrie, Joanne, "Table 1: Consequence of inadequate and excessive intake of selected nutrients," in *Away-From-Home Foods Increasingly Important to Quality of American Diet,* Economic Research Service, U.S. Department of Agriculture, Food and Drug Administration, Agricultural Information Bulletin # 749, 2000

needs of practically all healthy persons in a specific age (called life stage) and gender group. Derived from the EAR, the RDA can change allowances to permit variation within a particular group.

- Adequate Intake (AI)—the recommended intake of a nutrient where no RDA exists. AIs are established when sufficient scientific evidence is not available to estimate an average requirement. For example, AIs have been set for infants through one year of age, using as the standard the average observed nutrient intake of populations of healthy breast-feeding infants.

- Tolerable Upper Intake Level (TUIL)—the maximum intake unlikely to pose risks of adverse health effects in almost all healthy individuals in a specific group. Due to the popular use of dietary supplements and food fortification, the NAS, for the first time, sets these maximum-level guidelines to prevent overconsumption of a nutrient.

The Institute of Medicine will issue DRIs for seven nutrient groups:

- Calcium, vitamin D, phosphorus, magnesium, and fluoride.

- Folate (folic acid) and other B vitamins (thiamin, niacin, and riboflavin).

- Antioxidants, such as vitamins C and E and selenium.

- Macronutrients (protein, fat, and carbohydrate).

- Trace elements, such as iron and zinc.

- Electrolytes and water.

- Other food components, such as fiber and phytoestrogens.

In August 1997 the Institute of Medicine released the first of the new DRIs for calcium, phosphorus, magnesium, vitamin D, and fluoride, folates, B vitamins, and several other vitamins. Table 3.5 illustrates Dietary Reference Intakes for select nutrients, and Table 3.6 presents Recommended Daily Intakes (used by the Food and Drug Administration) for some dietary compounds.

VITAMINS

Vitamins are organic (carbon-containing) substances derived from animals or plants that are necessary in small amounts for growth and maintenance of life. Together with minerals, they are called micronutrients because, compared to macronutrients (carbohydrate, protein, fat, and water), they are needed in relatively small amounts.

The effects of vitamins have been understood on some level for thousands of years. In about 1500 AD, some people realized that eating certain foods could affect the development of certain diseases. From this, theories developed as to which foods cured deficiency diseases such as scurvy, rickets, and night blindness. Eventually vitamins were isolated and their biochemical functions and required amounts determined. Traditionally scientists have recognized 13 vitamins as needed by the human body. In April 1998 the National Academy of Sciences added the vitamin choline to the new DRIs.

TABLE 3.5

Dietary reference intakes: Recommended levels for individual intake[a]

Life-Stage Group	Calcium mg/day	Phosphorus mg/day	Magnesium mg/day	Vitamin D μg[b]	Flouride mg/day	Thiamine mg/day	Riboflavin mg/day	Niacin[d] mg/day	Vitamin B mg/day	Folate[e] μg/day	Vitamin B 12 μg/day	Pantothenic Acid mg/day	Biotin μg/day	Choline[f] mg/day
Infants														
0–6 mo.	210*	100*	30*	5*	0.01*	0.2*	0.3*	2*	0.1*	65*	0.4*	1.7*	5*	125*
7–12 mo.	270*	275*	75*	5*	0.5*	0.3*	0.4*	4*	0.3*	80*	0.5*	1.8*	6*	150*
Children														
1–3 y	500*	460	80	5*	0.7*	0.5	0.5	6	0.5	150	0.9	2*	8*	200*
4–8 y	800*	500	130	5*	1*	0.6	0.6	8	0.6	200	1.2	3*	12*	250*
Males														
9–13 y	1,300*	1,250	240	5*	2*	0.9	0.9	12	1	300	1.8	4*	20*	375*
14–18 y	1,300*	1,250	410	5*	3*	1.2	1.3	16	1.3	400	2.4	5*	25*	550*
19–30 y	1,000*	700	400	5*	4*	1.2	1.3	16	1.3	400	2.4	5*	30*	550*
31–50 y	1,000*	700	420	5*	4*	1.2	1.3	16	1.3	400	2.4	5*	30*	550*
51–70 y	1,200*	700	420	10*	4*	1.2	1.3	16	1.7	400	2.4 (g)	5*	30*	550*
>70 y	1,200*	700	420	15*	4*	1.2	1.3	16	1.7	400	2.4 (g)	5*	30*	550*
Females														
9–13 y	1,300*	1,250	240	5*	2*	0.9	0.9	12	1	300	1.8	4*	20*	375*
14–18 y	1,300*	1,250	360	5*	3*	1	1	14	1.2	400 (h)	2.4	5*	25*	400*
19–30 y	1,000*	700	310	5*	3*	1.1	1.1	14	1.3	400 (h)	2.4	5*	30*	425*
31–50 y	1,000*	700	320	5*	3*	1.1	1.1	14	1.3	400 (h)	2.4	5*	30*	425*
51–70 y	1,200*	700	320	10*	3*	1.1	1.1	14	1.5	400	2.4 (g)	5*	30*	425*
>70 y	1,200*	700	320	15*	3*	1.1	1.1	14	1.5	400	2.4 (g)	5*	30*	425*
Pregnancy														
<18 y	1,300*	1,250	400	5*	3*	1.4	1.4	18	1.9	600 (i)	2.6	6*	30*	450*
19–30 y	1,000*	700	350	5*	3*	1.4	1.4	18	1.9	600 (i)	2.6	6*	30*	450*
31–50 y	1,000*	700	360	5*	3*	1.4	1.4	18	1.9	600 (i)	2.6	6*	30*	450*
Lactation														
<18 y	1,300*	1,250	360	5*	3*	1.5	1.6	17	2	500	2.8	7*	35*	550*
19–30 y	1,000*	700	310	5*	3*	1.5	1.6	17	2	500	2.8	7*	35*	550*
31–50 y	1,000*	700	320	5*	3*	1.5	1.6	17	2	500	2.8	7*	35*	550*

(a) Recommended Dietary Allowances (RDAs) are presented in bold type and Adequate Intakes (AIs) in ordinary type followed by an asterisk (*). RDAs and AIs may both be used as goals for individual intake. RDAs are set to meet the needs of almost all (97% to 98%) individuals in a group. For healthy breast-fed infants, the AI is the mean intake. The AI for other life-stage and gender groups is believed to cover needs of all individuals in the group, but lack of data or uncertainty in the data prevent being able to specify with confidence the percentage of persons covered by this intake. Source: The Natural Academy of Sciences, Copyright 1998.

(b) As cholecalciferol. 1 μg cholecalciferol = 40 IU vitamin D.

(c) In the absence of adequate esposure to sunlight.

(d) As niacin equivalents (NE). 1 mg niacin = 60 mg tryptothan; 0 to 6 mo = preformed niacin (not NE).

(e) As dietary folate equivalent (DFE). 1 DFE = 1 μg food folate = 0.6 μg folic acid (from fortified food or supplement) consumed with food = 0.5 μg synthetic (supplemental) folic acid taken on an empty stomach.

(f) Although AIs have been set for choline, there are few data to assess whether a dietary supply of choline is needed at all stages of the life cycle, and it may be that the choline requirement can be met by endogenous synthesis at some of these stages.

(g) Because 10% to 30% of older people may malabsorb food-bound vitamin B-12, it is advisable for those older than 50 years to meet their RDA mainly by consuming foods fortified with vitamin B-12 or a supplement containing vitamin B-12.

(h) In view of evidence linking folate intake with neural tube defects in the fetus, it is recommended that all women capable of becoming pregnant consume 400 μg synthetic folic acid from fortified foods and/or supplements in addition to intake of food folate from a varied diet.

(i) It is assumed that women will continue consuming 400 μg folic acid until their pregnancy is confirmed and they enter prenatal care, which ordinarily occurs after the end of the periconceptional period- the critical time for formation of the neural tube.

SOURCE: "Dietary Reference Intakes (RDIs)," Food and Nutrition Board, National Academy of Sciences, Washington, D.C., 1998

TABLE 3.6

Recommended daily intake of selected dietary components

Gender and age	Dietary Recommendations							
	Calories[1]	Fat[2]	Saturated fat[2]	Cholesterol[3]	Sodium[4]	Fiber[5]	Calcium[1]	Iron[1]
	Calories	Percent	Percent	Mg	Mg	Grams	Mg	Mg
Children								
2–3	1,300	≤ 30	< 10	300	2,400	Age+5/day	800	10
4–6	1,800	≤ 30	< 10	300	2,400	Age+5/day	800	10
7–10	2,000	≤ 30	< 10	300	2,400	Age+5/day	800	10
Males								
11–14	2,500	≤ 30	< 10	300	2,400	Age+5/day	1,200	12
15–18	3,000	≤ 30	< 10	300	2,400	Age+5/day	1,200	12
19–20	2,900	≤ 30	< 10	300	2,400	Age+5/day	1,200	10
21–24	2,900	≤ 30	< 10	300	2,400	11.5/1,000 calories	1,200	10
25–50	2,900	≤ 30	< 10	300	2,400	11.5/1,000 calories	800	10
51+	2,300	≤ 30	< 10	300	2,400	11.5/1,000 calories	800	10
Females								
11–14	2,200	≤ 30	< 10	300	2,400	Age+5/day	1,200	15
15–18	2,000	≤ 30	< 10	300	2,400	Age+5/day	1,200	15
19–20	2,000	≤ 30	< 10	300	2,400	Age+5/day	1,200	15
21–24	2,000	≤ 30	< 10	300	2,400	11.5/1,000 calories	1,200	15
25–50	2,000	≤ 30	< 10	300	2,400	11.5/1,000 calories	800	15
51+	1,900	≤ 30	< 10	300	2,400	11.5/1,000 calories	800	10

[1] National Research Council's *Recommended Dietary Allowances.*
[2] U.S. Department of Health and Human Services and U.S. Department of Agriculture's *1995 Nutrition and Your Health: Dietary Guidelines for Americans.*
[3] U.S. Food and Drug Administration's (FDA) Daily Values (Kurtzweil).
[4] National Research Council's *Diet and Health* (National Academy Press, 1989).
[5] American Health Foundation for "age plus 5" per day (Williams) and FDA's Daily Value for 11.5 grams per 1,000 calories (Kurtzweil).

SOURCE: Lin, Biing-Hwan, Fazio, Elizabeth and Guthrie, Joanne, "Table 4: Recommended daily intake of selected dietary components," in *Away-From-Home Foods Increasingly Important to Quality of American Diet,* Economic Research Service, U.S. Department of Agriculture, Food and Drug Administration, Agricultural Information Bulletin # 749, 2000

Vitamins are either fat-soluble or water-soluble. Fat-soluble vitamins (A, D, E, and K), as their name suggests, dissolve in fat. They can be stored in the body for long periods and not excreted, leading to toxicity if a person takes large doses of supplements. Because they do not dissolve in water, fat-soluble vitamins are generally retained in foods during preparation. Vitamin C and the eight B-complex vitamins—thiamin, riboflavin, niacin, pyridoxine, cobalamin, pantothenic acid, biotin, and folate (folic acid)—are water-soluble. They are more likely to be destroyed during food preparation. Since the body excretes excess quantities of these vitamins, dangerous buildups in the body are unlikely.

Today researchers have moved beyond the link between vitamins and deficiency diseases to a greater recognition of the role of vitamins in disease prevention. American scientists no longer emphasize getting enough vitamins to prevent deficiency diseases, such as scurvy or rickets. Instead, studies focus on the role of vitamins in preventing cancer, heart disease, cataracts, and other chronic diseases.

VITAMINS AS ANTIOXIDANTS

In order to sustain life, the body uses oxygen to convert food into energy in a process called metabolism. As the body cells consume oxygen, they produce unstable oxygen molecules, known as free radicals. These unstable molecules, which have one or more unpaired electrons, are drawn toward molecules in cells in order to combine with their electrons. In this ongoing process, enough molecules may be damaged to cause cell death. Scientists believe that free radicals may cause the development of cancer through this destructive behavior and may even be responsible for the development of heart disease.

Environmental factors, including ultraviolet light, radiation, cigarette smoke, alcohol, and certain pollutants, such as ozone, also produce free radicals in the body. The body makes its own antioxidants that combine with free radicals, neutralizing their harmful actions. Scientists, however, believe that there are more free radicals than the body can handle. A group of nutrients found in food—mainly vitamins C and E and carotenoids—have been found to act as antioxidants, helping the body's defense against free radicals.

Vitamin C

A special report, "Can Antioxidants Save Your Life?" (*University of California at Berkeley Wellness Letter,* vol. 14, issue 10, July 1998), describes how vitamins C and E and carotenoids function as antioxidants. Vitamin C (also

TABLE 3.7

TABLE 3.8

Fruits and vegetables recommended by the National Cancer Institute

In selecting your daily intake of fruits and vegetables, the National Cancer Institute recommends choosing:

- At least one serving of a vitamin A-rich fruit or vegetable a day.
- At least one serving of a vitamin C-rich fruit or vegetable a day.
- At least one serving of a high-fiber fruit or vegetable a day.
- Several serving of cruciferous vegetables a week. Studies suggest that these vegetables may offer additional protection against certain cancers, although further research is needed.

High in Vitamin A*	High in Vitamin C*	High in Fiber or Good Source of Fiber*	Cruciferous Vegetables
apricots	apricots	apple	bok choy
cantaloupe	broccoli	banana	broccoli
carrots	brussels sprouts	blackberries	brussels sprouts
kale, collards	cabbage	blueberries	cabbage
leaf lettuce	cantaloupe	brussel sprouts	cauliflower
mango	cauliflower	carrots	
mustard greens	chili peppers	cherries	
pumpkin	collards	cooked beans and peas	
romaine lettuce	grapefruit	(kidney, navy, lima,	
spinach	honeydew melon	and pinto beans, lentils	
sweet potato	kiwi fruit	black-eyed peas)	
winter squash	mango	dates	
(acorn, hubbard)	mustard greens	figs	
	orange	grapefruit	
	orange juice	kiwi fruit	
	pineapple	orange	
	plum	pear	
	potato with skin	prunes	
	spinach	raspberries	
	strawberries	spinach	
	bell peppers	strawberries	
	tangerine	sweet potato	
	tomatoes		
	watermelon		

*Based on FDA's food labeling regulations.

SOURCE: Paula Kurtzweil, "Fruits and Vegetables: Eating Your Way to Five a Day," reprinted from *FDA Consumer,* March 1997, revised August 1998

Which fruits and vegetables provide the most nutrients?

The lists below show which fruits and vegetables are the best sources of vitamin A (carotenoids), vitamin C, folate, and potassium. Eat at least 2 servings of fruits and at least 3 servings of vegetables each day:

Sources of vitamin A (carotenoids)
- Orange vegetables like carrots, sweet potatoes, pumpkin
- Dark-green leafy vegetables such as spinach, collards, turnip greens
- Orange fruits like mango, cantaloupe, apricots
- Tomatoes

Sources of vitamin C
- Citrus fruits and juices, kiwi fruit, strawberries, cantaloupe
- Broccoli, peppers, tomatoes, cabbage, potatoes
- Leafy greens such as romaine lettuce, turnip greens, spinach

Sources of folate
- Cooked dry beans and peas, peanuts
- Oranges, orange juice
- Dark-green leafy vegetables like spinach and mustard greens, romaine lettuce
- Green peas

Sources of potassium
- Baked white or sweet potato, cooked greens (such as spinach), winter (orange) squash
- Bananas, plantains, dried fruits such as apricots and prunes, orange juice
- Cooked dry beans (such as baked beans) and lentils

Note: Read nutrition facts labels for product-specific information, especially for processed fruits and vegetables.

SOURCE: "Which Fruits and Vegtables Provide the Most Nutients? " in *Dietary Guidelines for Americans, 2000,* U.S. Department of Agruculture, Washington, D.C.,2000

known as ascorbic acid) not only fights free radicals, but also interferes with the formation of nitrosamines (cancer-causing compounds) from nitrites found in such foods as hot dogs, ham, and sausages. Low vitamin C in the diet has been linked to an increased risk of stomach, esophagus, lung, breast, cervical, colon, and bladder cancer.

Vitamin C's antioxidant action can also help prevent cataracts. Scientists have found that eye fluids contain large amounts of vitamin C and other antioxidants, causing them to believe that vitamin C may protect the eye from free radicals produced by sunlight. Moreover, vitamin C plays an important role in preventing heart disease and birth defects.

VITAMIN C'S OTHER FUNCTIONS. Scurvy, the disease most associated with vitamin C deficiency, is rare in the United States and other developed countries due to adequate consumption of fresh fruits and vegetables, the highest sources of this vitamin. Vitamin C also performs other important functions in the body. It helps in the formation of collagen (connective tissue) and bones, the absorption of iron and excretion of lead, and the production of certain antibodies.

Vitamin C stimulates the production of epinephrine (formerly called adrenalin) and norepinephrine (noradrenalin), hormones released in times of danger to strengthen and prepare a person for "fight or flight." Vitamin C also helps convert folic acid to its active form and "regenerates" vitamin E oxidized during cell metabolism. Scientists describe "regeneration" as the process by which an antioxidant revives another antioxidant that has been oxidized (combined with a free radical). Nutritionists advise consumers to get vitamin C from fruits and vegetables. (See Table 3.7.)

Vitamin E

Scientists at the University of California at Berkeley discovered vitamin E in 1922. During the 1990s, a growing body of research worldwide suggested that vitamin E may prevent heart disease; reduce the risk of cancer, including prostate cancer; delay aging; and prevent or postpone the development of cataracts. Vitamin E may also help reduce the symptoms of Parkinson's disease, a degenerative disorder of the brain's nerve centers.

University of California at Berkeley researchers believe vitamin E may reduce the risk of heart disease because it prevents the oxidation of low-density lipoprotein (LDL, "bad") cholesterol. When LDL cholesterol is attacked, or oxidized, by free radicals, it is predisposed to accelerate the buildup of plaque, a condition called atherosclerosis that may result in a heart attack or a stroke. Vitamin E traps free radicals quickly because it is carried in the bloodstream by LDL.

Carotenoids

Carotenoids are the pigments that give plants their red, orange, and yellow colors. Once valued only as provitamins, or precursors of vitamin A (they can be converted by the liver to vitamin A as needed), these compounds have been found to possess nutritional values of their own. Scientists have discovered more than 600 carotenoids; the body can convert about 50 into active vitamin A. Beta-carotene is the best known of the group but other important carotenoids include alpha-carotene, gamma-carotene, beta-cryptoxanthin, lycopene, lutein, and zeaxanthin. Table 3.8 shows fruits and vegetables that are good sources of different carotenoids.

There is growing evidence that carotenoids may play an important role against such diseases as cancer and heart disease. Lycopene, found in tomatoes and tomato products, such as pizza sauce and ketchup, has been linked to the prevention of prostate cancer. Like vitamin E, it prevents the oxidation of LDL cholesterol. Alpha-carotene, found abundantly in carrots, is associated with reduced risk of lung cancer. Cryptoxanthin, found in many orange-colored fruits, may decrease the risk of cervical cancer.

CONTROVERSIES OVER BETA-CAROTENE. Beta-carotene, the most popular of carotenoids, is said to boost the immune system, partly due to its antioxidant activity. It has also been linked to decreased risk of lung and oral cancers. However, two large clinical trials sponsored by the National Cancer Institute (NCI) of the National Institutes of Health (NIH) questioned the potential health benefits of beta-carotene.

The first study involved a collaboration between the NCI and the National Public Health Institute of Finland (the results of the study were released in 1994). The purpose of the *Alpha-Tocopherol, Beta-Carotene Cancer Prevention Trial* (ATBC Trial) was to determine if certain supplements would prevent lung cancer and other cancers in a group of over 29,000 male smokers in Finland. After five to eight years, 18 percent more lung cancers were diagnosed, and 8 percent more overall deaths occurred in the study participants taking beta-carotene.

The second study, the *Beta Carotene and Retinol Efficacy Trial* (CARET) was conducted to find out if a combination of beta-carotene and vitamin A would prevent lung and other cancers in men and women who were smokers or former smokers, as well as in men exposed to asbestos. In 1996, after an average of four years of taking the supplements, the over 18,000 participants were told to stop taking them. About 28 percent more lung cancers were diagnosed, and 17 percent more deaths occurred in

CARET participants taking beta-carotene and vitamin A than those taking placebos. Both studies found no significant evidence of any benefit in taking beta-carotene.

The *Physicians' Health Study* (National Institutes of Health, Bethesda, Md, 1999), a 12-year study of 22,000 U.S. male physicians funded by NIH's National Heart, Lung, and Blood Institute, found no significant evidence of either benefits or harm from beta-carotene on cancer or heart disease.

The National Cancer Institute reported one consistent finding from the ATBC Trial and CARET—participants with the highest levels of serum (blood-borne) beta-carotene (obtained from consumption of foods containing beta-carotene), measured before the clinical trial, developed fewer lung cancers.

The NCI does not recommend that Americans take dietary supplements of beta-carotene. Rather, it recommends that those who wish to reduce their risk of cancer adopt a low-fat diet containing plenty of fruits, vegetables, and grains. It continues to stress its "Five-A-Day" program of eating five servings of fruits and vegetables daily. (See Table 3.7.)

FOLATE (FOLIC ACID)

Folate, or folacin, is a B vitamin added to many vitamin and mineral supplements in the form of folic acid. In its April 1998 report on Dietary Reference Intakes (DRIs), the Institute of Medicine recommended that all adult (14 and over) men and women include 400 micrograms of folate in their diets daily. (See Table 3.5.) The Institute claimed that, although folic acid can be found in many food items, such as enriched bread, pasta, flour, breakfast cereal, crackers, and rice, many Americans still do not take enough folic acid. Consequently, starting January 1998, the Food and Drug Administration required manufacturers of grain products to fortify their foods with folic acid.

Every year in the United States about 4,000 pregnancies are affected by neural tube defects. About 2,500 of these pregnancies involve infants born with the two most common neural tube defects—anencephaly (absence of a major part of the brain, skull, and scalp) or spina bifida (incomplete closure of the spinal column). These conditions result from the disruption of the fetus's central nervous system in the first month of pregnancy, when many women may not realize they are pregnant.

To reduce the risk of neural tube defects, the Institute of Medicine recommends that women capable of becoming pregnant should consume 400 micrograms of folic acid daily from fortified foods and/or supplements in addition to folate from a varied diet. For pregnant women, the Institute recommends 600 micrograms. (See Table 3.5.) However, the February 1999 *University of California*

TABLE 3.9

Food sources of folate

Food	Micrograms dietary folate equivalents	% DV*
Ready to eat cereal, fortified with 100% of the DV, 3/4 cup	400	100
Beef liver, cooked, braised, 3 oz	185	45
Cowpeas (blackeyes), immature, cooked, boiled, 1/2 cup	105	25
Breakfast cereals, fortified with 25% of the DV, 3/4 cup	100	25
Spinach, frozen, cooked, boiled,1/2 cup	100	25
Great Northern beans, boiled, 1/2 cup	90	20
Asparagus, boiled, 4 spears	85	20
Wheat germ, toasted, 1/4 cup	80	20
Orange juice, chilled, includes concentrate, 3/4 cup	70	20
Turnip greens, frozen, cooked, boiled, 1/2 cup	65	15
Vegetarian baked beans, canned, 1 cup	60	15
Spinach, raw, 1 cup	60	15
Green peas, boiled, 1/2 cup	50	15
Broccoli, chopped, frozen, cooked, 1/2 cup	50	15
Egg noodles, cooked, enriched, 1/2 cup	15	50
Rice, white, long-grain, parboiled, cooked, enriched, 1/2 cup	45	10
Avocado, raw, all varieties, sliced 1/2 c sliced	45	10
Peanuts, all types, dry roasted, 1 oz	40	10
Lettuce, romaine, shredded, 1/2 cup	40	10
Tomato juice, canned, 6 oz	35	10
Orange, all commercial varieties, fresh, 1 small	30	8
Bread, white, enriched, 1 slice	25	6
Egg, whole, raw, fresh, 1 large	25	6
Cantaloupe, raw, 1/4 medium	25	6
Papaya, raw, 1/2 c cubes	25	6
Banana, raw, 1 medium	20	6
Broccoli, raw, 1 spear (about 5 inches long)	20	6
Lettuce, iceberg, shredded,1/2 cup	15	4
Bread, whole wheat, 1 slice	15	4

* DV = Daily Value. DVs are reference numbers based on the Recommended Dietary Allowance (RDA). They were developed to help consumers determine if a food contains a lot or a little of a specific nutrient. The DV for folic acid is 400 micrograms (mcg). The percent DV (%DV) listed on the nutrition facts panel of food labels tells adults what percentage of the DV is provided by one serving. Percent DVs are based on a 2,000 calorie diet. Your Daily Values may be higher or lower depending on your calorie needs. Foods that provide lower percentages of the DV also contribute to a healthful diet.

SOURCE: "Table of Selected Food Sources of Folate" in *Facts About Dietary Supplements*, Clinical Nutrition Service, Office of Dietary Supplements, National Institutes of Health, Washington, D.C., 2000

TABLE 3.10

Knowledge and use of folic acid among women of childbearing age 1995 and 1998*

Characteristic	1995	1998
Knowledge		
Heard of folic acid	52%	68%
Knew folic acid can help prevent birth defects	5%	13%
Knew folic acid should be taken before pregnancy	2%	7%
Behavior		
Take folic acid daily (nonpregnant women)	25%	29%
Take folic acid daily (all women)	28%	32%
Source of knowledge		
Magazine/newspaper	35%	31%
Radio/television	10%	23%
Health-care provider	13%	19%

*The margin of error for estimates based on the total sample size was ±3%.

SOURCE: "Knowledge, behavior, and source of knowledge regarding folic acid among childbearing-aged women--United States, 1995 and 1998" in "Knowledge and Use of Folic Acid by Women of Childbearing Age—United States, 1995 and 1998," *Morbidity and Mortality Weekly Report*, Vol. 48, No. 16, April 30, 1999, Centers for Disease Control and Prevention, Atlanta, GA

48, no. 16, April 30, 1999), reported that a 1998 nationwide survey by the March of Dimes Birth Defects Foundation found that over two-thirds (68 percent) of women ages 18 to 45 (prime childbearing years) had heard of or read about folic acid, up from 52 percent in 1995. (See Table 3.10.)

In 1998, 13 percent of all respondents knew folic acid can help prevent birth defects, up from 5 percent in 1995, and 7 percent knew folic acid should be taken before pregnancy, up from 2 percent in 1995. In 1998, among women not pregnant at the time of the survey, 29 percent were taking a vitamin supplement containing folic acid, compared to 25 percent in 1995. Nearly one-third (32 percent) of all women reported taking a vitamin supplement containing folic acid, compared to 28 percent in 1995. (See Table 3.10) Women the most likely to take vitamin supplements containing folic acid daily included those ages 25 to 45 (34 percent), college graduates (40 percent), and higher-income women (for example, 38 percent among those with annual household income of $50,000 or more).

The proportion of women who obtained folic acid information from magazine or newspaper articles decreased from 35 percent in 1995 to 31 percent in 1998. On the other hand, the proportion that learned about folic acid from radio or television increased from 10 to 23 percent, while the proportion who learned from health-care providers rose from 13 to 19 percent during the same time period. (See Table 3.10.)

at Berkeley Wellness Letter (vol. 15, issue 5) reported that a number of studies show folic acid in vitamin supplements and folic acid used to fortify foods are better absorbed by the body than the folate naturally occurring in food. Table 3.9 shows some good sources of folate.

Knowledge and Use of Folic Acid

The Centers for Disease Control and Prevention (CDC), in "Knowledge and Use of Folic Acid by Women of Childbearing Age—United States, 1995 and 1998" (*Morbidity and Mortality Weekly Report,* vol.

DIETARY FIBER

For centuries, human beings have recognized that dietary fiber is beneficial to the normal functioning of the digestive system. Formerly called roughage or bulk, fiber has always been considered invaluable in preventing constipation. Dr. Victor Herbert, in "Dietary Fiber" (*Total Nutrition: The Only Guide You'll Ever Need,* Mount Sinai School of Medicine, St. Martin's Press, New York, 1995), defines dietary fiber as "the sum of the unabsorbable crude fiber (mainly cellulose and lignin) remaining in the colon after digestion, plus the available (fermentable) fiber."

Dietary fibers are either soluble or insoluble:

- Soluble fibers—fibers that combine with water, forming gels. They include pectin, guar, mucilages, and most hemicelluloses. Foods containing soluble fibers include oat bran, barley, dried beans, other legumes, and some vegetables and fruits.

- Insoluble fibers—as their name suggests, fibers that do not dissolve in water. Therefore, they pass through the digestive tract, reduced in size by chewing but unchanged. These include cellulose, some hemicelluloses, and lignin (which is found in the woody part of vegetables and fruit seeds). Whole-grain products, wheat bran, and the skins of fruits and vegetables contain insoluble fibers.

A Lot to Learn

Ruth Papazian, in "Bulking Up Fiber's Healthful Reputation" (*FDA Consumer,* September 1998), reported that, in 1996 when Americans were asked which foods—lettuce, asparagus, navy beans, brown rice, oatmeal—are the best sources of cholesterol-lowering soluble fibers, 60 percent chose navy beans and 75 percent chose oatmeal (correct answers). However, nearly half mistakenly identified lettuce (46 percent) and asparagus (48 percent) and almost two-thirds (64 percent) incorrectly chose brown rice as sources of soluble fibers that help reduce blood cholesterol. (See Figure 3.3.)

No Specific Dietary Allowance

No Recommended Dietary Allowances (RDAs) currently exist for dietary fiber. The American Heart Association urges consumers to increase their intake to 25 to 30 grams of dietary fiber daily, although the typical American consumes only about 11 grams a day. The U.S. Food and Drug Administration (FDA), recognizing the growing numbers of studies showing the health benefits of fiber, now requires the inclusion of fiber on the Nutrition Facts food labels that list other important nutrients. The Daily Values on food labels recommend a dietary fiber intake of 25 grams for individuals consuming 2,000 calories daily and 30 grams for those consuming 2,500 calories. In addition, the FDA has approved four health claims for dietary fiber on food labels. According to Ruth Papazian, recent studies show that dietary fiber may play a role in reducing the risk of certain cancers, diabetes, digestive disorders, and heart disease.

FIGURE 3.3

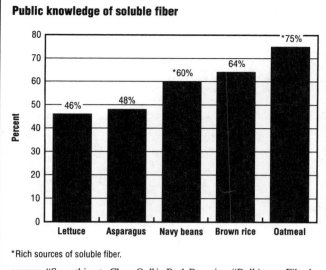

Public knowledge of soluble fiber

*Rich sources of soluble fiber.

SOURCE: "Something to Chew On" in Ruth Papazian, "Bulking up Fiber's Healthful Reputation," *FDA Consumer,* July-August 1997, U.S. Food and Drug Administration, Washington, D.C.

Dietary Fiber and Health

CONSTIPATION AND DIVERTICULOSIS. The role of fiber in preventing constipation has long been recognized. Insoluble fiber, capable of absorbing as much as 15 times its weight in water, adds to the water-holding capacity of large intestine contents, increasing stool bulk. The passage of stool through the digestive track is expedited, thus preventing and relieving constipation.

Dietary fiber may also help reduce the risk of diverticulosis, a condition where diverticula, or small abnormal pockets, form in the wall of the colon (the main part of the large intestine). These sac-like protrusions along the inner lining of the large intestine are usually caused by straining during bowel movement or simply by aging. Kathleen Meister, in *Dietary Fiber* (American Council on Science and Health, New York, December 1996) reports that "one-third of all North Americans over the age of 45 and two-thirds of all persons over the age of 85 have diverticula in their colons." A number of studies have found that a diet high in fiber may prevent diverticulosis.

While most cases of diverticulosis cause no symptoms, the diverticula may get inflamed, causing a condition called diverticulitis, characterized by fever and pain. Hospitalization and surgery may be needed, especially if perforations occur. Dietary fiber is not part of the treatment of diverticulitis.

CANCER. Scientists who have studied the relationship between a high-fiber diet and a lower incidence of colon cancer believe that insoluble fiber not only adds bulk to stool but also dilutes carcinogens (cancer-causing sub-

TABLE 3.11

Sources of dietary fiber

Rich Sources of Dietary Fiber (4 or more grams of fiber per serving)		
Breads and Cereals	Cereals with 4 or more grams fiber per serving (check product Nutrition Facts Label)	1/3 – 1/2 cup (varies)
Legumes (cooked)	Beans, brown	1/2 cup
	Beans, kidney	1/2 cup
	Beans, large lima	1/2 cup
	Beans, navy	1/2 cup
	Beans, pinto	1/2 cup
	Beans, white	1/2 cup
	Lentils	1/2 cup
	Peas, black-eyed	1/2 cup
Vegetables	Artichoke, cooked	1 each
Fruits	Blackberries	1/2 cup
	Prunes, dried	4 each
	Raspberries	1/2 cup

Moderately Rich Sources of Dietary Fiber (1 to 3 grams of fiber per serving)		
Breads	Bagel, 3.5" diameter	1 each
	Bread; whole wheat, cracked wheat, pumpernickel, or rye	1 slice
	Corn bread	2" square
	Crackers, whole wheat	4 each
	Muffin; bran, blueberry, cornmeal, or English	1 each
Cereals	Cereals with 1-3 grams of fiber per serving (check product Nutrition Facts Label)	1/2 cup (varies)
	Bran, rice, or wheat	2 tablespoons
	Wheat germ	2 tablespoons
Fruits	Apple, 2 3/4" diameter	1 each
	Applesauce	1/2 cup
	Apricots, canned	1/2 cup
	Banana	1 each
	Cherries, canned or fresh	1/2 cup
	Cranberries, fresh	1/2 cup
	Dates, whole	3 each
	Figs, fresh, medium	2 each
	Fruit cocktail, canned	1/2 cup
	Grapefruit	1 half
	Kiwi fruit	1 each
	Orange, 2 5/8" diameter	1 each
	Peaches, canned	1/2 cup
	Peaches, fresh	1 each
	Pears, canned	1/2 cup
	Pears, fresh	1/2 each
	Plum, medium, 2 1/8" diameter	1 each
	Raisins	1/4 cup
	Strawberries, fresh	1/2 cup
	Tangerine	1 each

Vegetables	Bean sprouts, raw	1/2 cup
	Beets, diced, canned	1/2 cup
	Broccoli, chopped, frozen, boiled	1/2 cup
	Brussels sprouts	1/2 cup
	Cabbage, cooked	1/2 cup
	Carrots	1/2 cup
	Cauliflower	1/2 cup
	Corn	1/2 cup
	Eggplant	1/2 cup
	Kale, boiled	1/2 cup
	Okra, frozen, boiled	1/2 cup
	Potatoes, baked or mashed	1/2 cup
	Spinach	1/2 cup
	Squash, winter or summer	1/2 cup
	Sweet potatoes	1/2 cup
	Tomatoes, canned	1/2 cup
	Turnip greens	1/2 cup
	Yams	1/2 cup
	Zucchini, cooked	1/2 cup
Miscellaneous	Almonds	2 tablespoons
	Flour, whole wheat	2 tablespoons
	Peanuts	2 tablespoons
	Popcorn, popped	1 cup

Low Sources of Dietary Fiber (less than 1 gram of fiber per serving)		
Breads and Cereals	Bread; white, raisin, or pita	1 slice or 1 each
	Cereals with less than 1 gram of fiber per serving (check product Nutrition Facts Label)	1/2 cup (varies)
	Crackers, saltine	4 each
	Crackers, graham	2 each
	Rice, white	1/2 cup
	Roll, white dinner	1 each
Fruits	Cantaloupe	1/6 each
	Grapes, Thompson seedless	1/2 cup
	Juices, grape, orange, etc.	1/2 cup
	Mandarin oranges	1/2 cup
	Watermelon	1 cup
Vegetables	Asparagus, cooked	3 spears
	Beans, green	1/2 cup
	Chestnuts, water	1/2 cup
	Lettuce, iceberg, chopped	1 cup
	Mushrooms, canned	1/2 cup
	Mustard greens, fresh	1/2 cup
	Onions, chopped, raw	1/4 cup
	Pepper, sweet green	1/2 cup
Miscellaneous	Flour, white	2 tablespoons

SOURCE: "Rich Sources of Dietary Fiber," "Moderately Rich Sources of Dietary Fiber," and "Low Sources of Dietary Fiber" in Janice R. Hermann, *Dietary Fiber,* Oklahoma Cooperative Extension Service, Division of Agricultural Sciences and Natural Resources, Oklahoma State University, Stillwater, OK, May 1999

stances) in the stool. In addition, since stool bulk helps decrease its travel time through the digestive tract, it thereby reduces the colon's exposure to carcinogens.

Some studies suggest there may be a correlation between high-fiber intake and a reduced risk of breast cancer. Papazian reports, "In the early stages, some breast tumors are stimulated by excess amounts of estrogen circulating in the bloodstream." Some scientists think that dietary fiber may combine with estrogen in the intestine, reducing excess estrogen levels in the bloodstream and thus preventing further growth of breast tumors.

HEART DISEASE. There is some evidence that a high intake of dietary fiber, especially soluble fiber, can lower low-density lipoprotein (LDL) blood cholesterol. LDL, also called "bad cholesterol," is responsible for forming the plaque that contributes to coronary heart disease (CHD). As soluble fiber passes through the digestive tract, it links with "bad cholesterol" and helps remove it from the body.

Coronary heart disease is the leading killer of women. Alicja Wolk et al., in "Long-Term Intake of Dietary Fiber and Decreased Risk of Coronary Heart Disease Among Women" (*The Journal of the American Medical Association,* vol. 281, no. 21, June 2, 1999), examined 68,782 women ages 37 to 64 who were enrolled in the 10-year longitudinal *Nurses' Health Study.*

The researchers found that, of the three sources of dietary fiber—cereals, fruits, and vegetables—only cereal fiber was strongly linked to decreased risk of CHD in women. Consumption of cold cereal five or more times per week, compared to nonconsumption, was linked to a 19 percent lower risk of CHD. Consumption of oatmeal (soluble fiber) was associated with a 29 percent lower risk of CHD. Eating fruit and vegetable fibers was not significantly related to the risk of CHD. Similar results have been found in studies among men.

DIABETES. In the late 1980s and early 1990s, when it was thought that dietary fiber (particularly soluble fiber) might help regulate blood sugar, health professionals prescribed a daily dietary fiber intake of up to 40 grams for diabetics. However, further research has shown that an unusually large amount of fiber is needed to control blood sugar, and that not all soluble fibers achieve the same antidiabetic result. In 1994 the American Dietetic Association recommended that diabetics should consume the same amount of dietary fibers as nondiabetics.

Measuring the amount of fiber in food can be difficult because scientists do not agree on which method is best. The amount of fiber can vary by as much as 30 percent depending on the method of analysis. Oklahoma State University's Division of Agricultural Sciences provides a listing of rich and moderate sources of fiber. (See Table 3.11.)

Caution in Using Dietary Fiber

Although Americans are encouraged to increase their intake of dietary fiber, they should not necessarily use dietary supplements to boost their intake. In fact, nutritionists and other health professionals generally discourage the use of dietary supplements. Experts also recommend that fiber should come from a variety of foods, be increased gradually, and be eaten throughout the day instead of during one sitting. Some people experience gas pains, bloating, and even diarrhea after eating a large amount of fiber. Excessive fiber consumption may also prevent the absorption of some minerals, such as calcium, zinc, and iron.

Fiber in Children's Diets

Kathleen Meister, in *Dietary Fiber,* warns against adding too much fiber to children's diets. High-fiber foods tend to be bulky and low calorie, and children need many calories for normal growth and development. In addition, fiber may fill them up quickly, leaving little room for other foods. As with adults, children cannot

TABLE 3.12

Composition of fats

Kind of fat	%Saturated	%Poly	%Mono
Canola oil	6	32	62
Safflower oil	10	77	13
Sunflower oil	11	69	20
Corn oil	13	62	25
Olive oil	14	9	77
Soybean oil	15	61	24
Margarine (tub)	17	34	24
Peanut oil	18	33	49
Cottonseed oil	27	54	19
Chicken fat	31	22	47
Lard	41	12	47
Beef fat	52	4	44
Palm kernal oil	81	2	11
Coconut oil	92	2	6

SOURCE: *Composition of Foods,* U.S. Department of Agriculture, Washington, D.C.

afford to lose the minerals that may be combined with unabsorbed fiber excreted from the body. The American Academy of Pediatrics recommends 0.5 grams of dietary fiber for each kilogram of a child's body weight, while the American Health Foundation recommends that a child age three and over have a dietary fiber intake equivalent to his or her age plus 5 grams daily.

DIETARY FATS AND CHOLESTEROL

All dietary fats are mixtures of saturated and unsaturated fatty acids. Fatty acids are the building blocks of dietary fats. Fatty acids are classified as saturated or unsaturated, based on their chemical composition, that is, the number of hydrogen atoms they contain.

Saturated fatty acids contain the most hydrogen atoms—in other words, they are "saturated" with hydrogen. Saturated fats, found in meat, egg yolks, and whole-milk dairy products, are generally solid at room temperature. Three vegetable fats—coconut oil, palm oil, and palm kernel oil—are very high in saturated fats. (See Table 3.12.)

Unsaturated fats, which are missing hydrogen atoms, are generally liquid at room temperature and are called oils. Plants and fish are the main sources of unsaturated fats. Unsaturated fats are classified as monounsaturated or polyunsaturated. Monounsaturated fats, such as olive, canola, and peanut oils, are missing a pair of hydrogen atoms, while polyunsaturated fats are missing two or more pairs of hydrogen atoms. Corn, soybean, safflower, and sesame seed oils are polyunsaturated fats. (See Table 3.12.)

Fats, Cholesterol, and Coronary Heart Disease

Health professionals recommend limiting fat intake to 30 percent or less of total daily calories and saturated fat intake to less than 10 percent of calories. The *Third National Health and Nutrition Examination Survey*

FIGURE 3.4

Example of cholesterol plaque buildup in a blood vessel

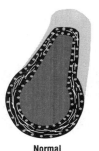 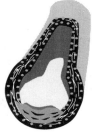 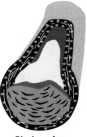

Normal   Buildup of cholesterol   Blockage from plaque formation

SOURCE: John Henkel, "The Plague of Plaque" in "Keeping Cholesterol Under Control," *FDA Consumer,* Jan-Feb, 1999.

TABLE 3.13

Cholesterol levels

Total blood cholesterol	Classification
Less than 200 mg/dL	Desirable
200-239 mg/dL	Borderline High
240 mg/dL and over	High
LDL cholesterol	**Classification**
Less than 130 mg/dL	Desirable
130-159 mg/dL	Borderline High
160 mg/dL or higher	High
HDL cholesterol	**Classification**
40-50 mg/dL(men)	Desirable
50-60 mg/dL (women)	Desirable
Less that 35 mg/dL	Low

SOURCE: National Heart, Lung, and Blood Institute, National Institutes of Health, Washington, D.C.

(NHANES III) found that Americans currently consume about 34 percent of their total calories as fat, with 12 percent of their calories provided by saturated fats.

Excess saturated fats in the diet have been found to elevate serum or blood cholesterol levels. High blood cholesterol has been recognized as a risk factor for coronary heart disease. Cholesterol is transported through the bloodstream by lipoproteins, a mixture of fats (lipids) and proteins. Excess blood cholesterol accumulates in the inner lining of the arterial walls, combining with fats and other substances to form plaque. (See Figure 3.4.) This condition is known as atherosclerosis. The arteries become narrowed due to these deposits, thereby reducing the flow of blood in these arteries. A thrombus or clot may form when blood flow is sluggish. If a clot forms where the plaque is located, the blood flow to the heart may be blocked, causing a heart attack. If blood flow to the brain is blocked, a stroke results.

Two lipoproteins are believed to play major roles in the amount of blood cholesterol. Low-density lipoprotein (LDL) contains most of the cholesterol found in the blood and is said to be responsible for the "bad cholesterol" that forms plaque. High-density lipoprotein (HDL) is believed to carry cholesterol from the arteries to the liver, where it is excreted from the body. According to the American Heart Association's *Heart and Stroke A-Z Guide* (2000), "Some experts believe HDL removes excess cholesterol from atherosclerotic plaques and thus slows their growth."

According to NHANES III, the average level of serum cholesterol in the U.S. population was 203 milligrams/deciliter (mg/dl). Between 1988 and 1994, 18.9 percent of the population had high serum cholesterol. Somewhat more females (20 percent) than males (17.5 percent) had high serum cholesterol, with 2 in 5 females age 55 and over having high serum cholesterol. The

National Cholesterol Education Program of the National Heart, Lung, and Blood Institute classifies the risk for coronary heart disease based on total serum cholesterol. Since the type of cholesterol also plays a major role in the risk of heart disease, the institute also provides a guideline. (See Table 3.13.)

Heart Benefits from Monounsaturated Fats

A number of studies have found that monounsaturated fats decrease bad cholesterol (LDL) levels and increase good cholesterol (HDL) levels. This does not mean, however, that people should indulge in large amounts of olive or canola oil, but that they would do better to choose monounsaturates over other fats, especially saturated fats.

A study in Lyon, France has again called attention to the diets of Mediterranean countries, which are noted for their high intake of fruits, vegetables, and breads, low consumption of meat, and the use of olive oil. The *Lyon Diet Heart Study* (*University of California at Berkeley Wellness Letter,* vol. 15, issue 8, May 1999) found that, among people from the Greek island of Crete who had had a heart attack in the six months prior to the study, a change in fat in their diet cut the risk of a second heart attack and the overall death rate by as much as 70 percent over the course of four years. Margarine made from canola (rapeseed) oil was used in place of other fats. Blood tests revealed a high concentration of a polyunsaturated fatty acid called alpha-linoleic acid, which is present in canola oil.

High concentrations of alpha-linoleic acid are found in few foods—canola, soybean, and flaxseed oils, as well as walnuts and the leafy, green vegetable purslane. Researchers believe that alpha-linoleic acid, a "short-chain" omega-3 fatty acid related to the "longer-chain" omega-3 fatty acid found in fish, may be capable of reducing blood clotting and heart-rhythm defects and of exerting an anti-inflammatory effect in blood vessels. The researchers, however, did not discount the beneficial effects the overall Mediterranean diet had on the patients' heart conditions.

Hydrogenation and Trans Fats

Food manufacturers use hydrogenation—the addition of hydrogen molecules to monounsaturated or polyunsaturated fatty acids—to prevent rancidity and promote better food textures. Fats normally break down when exposed to air and heat, becoming rancid. Hydrogenation stabilizes them, promoting freshness and helping extend their shelf lives. Hydrogenation also raises the melting point of oils, a characteristic useful in deep fat frying. Hydrogenation makes baked goods tender and flaky. Vegetable oils are often partially hydrogenated to create margarines and shortenings.

Food manufacturers use only as much hydrogenation as they need to achieve desired food tastes and textures. Foods that are partially hydrogenated still contain more unsaturated than saturated fats.

Trans fatty acids (trans fats) form when unsaturated fats become hydrogenated. Some studies have found that trans fats resulting from hydrogenation raise the blood levels of the "bad" LDL cholesterol, which increases the risk of heart disease. Until more studies confirm this, experts suggest that consumers use softer tub margarines instead of stick margarines and butter, and reduce their intake of fried foods.

Table 3.14 presents a comparison of saturated and unsaturated fat levels in certain foods. See Table 3.6 for recommended daily intakes for fat, saturated fat, and cholesterol.

CALCIUM

Calcium and Osteoporosis

The word osteoporosis means "porous bones." Osteoporosis is a disease that thins and weakens bones until they easily break. The bones of the hip, spine, and wrists are especially likely to break. It is called the "silent disease" because there are no visible symptoms of the weakening of bones. Physicians, however, can diagnose osteoporosis before fractures occur by using the bone density test.

The body's 206 bones are in a continual process of building, breaking down, and rebuilding. In the first few decades of life, rebuilding outpaces breakdown of bones, resulting in greater bone density and strength. The body forms most of its bone mass before puberty so that, during adolescence, about 75 to 85 percent of the skeleton is formed. Since the main mineral in bones is calcium, a growing body needs about 1,300 milligrams of calcium daily.

TABLE 3.14

Comparing saturated-fat content

Food category	Portion	Saturated fat content in (grams)
Cheese		
Regular Cheddar cheese	1 oz.	6.0
Low-fat Cheddar cheese*	1 oz.	1.2
Ground beef		
Regular ground beef	3 oz. cooked	7.2
Extra lean ground beef*	3 oz. cooked	5.3
Milk		
Whole milk	1 cup	5.1
Low-fat (1%) milk*	1 cup	1.6
Breads		
Croissant	1 medium	6.6
Bagel*	1 medium	0.1
Frozen desserts		
Regular ice cream	1/2 cup	4.5
Frozen yogurt*	1/2 cup	2.5
Table spreads		
Butter	1 tsp.	2.4
Soft margarine*	1 tsp.	0.7

Note: The food categories listed are among the major food sources of saturated fat for U.S. adults and children.

* Choice that is lower in saturated fat.

SOURCE: "A Comparison of Saturated Fat in Some Foods" in *Dietary Guidelines for Americans, 2000*, U.S. Department of Agriculture, Washington, D.C., 2000

Peak bone mass (maximum bone density and strength) is achieved somewhere between ages 20 and 30. After age 30, bones break down faster than they can be replaced. Nonetheless, the body continues to draw on the calcium in bones for functions such as muscle contraction. Bones that have not attained optimal mass tend to become thinner and more brittle with each calcium withdrawal.

Not all the causes of osteoporosis are fully known. It is recognized, however, that women lose bone mass at an accelerated rate after menopause. The ovaries produce lower levels of estrogen, which is responsible for protecting against bone loss. Some women begin to lose bone mass as early as age 35. Men also suffer bone loss but at a later age.

According to the National Osteoporosis Foundation, about 10 million people in the United States have osteoporosis, and another 18 million have low bone mass, putting them at increased risk for the disease. Osteoporosis is a threat to four out of five women.

Osteoporosis is responsible for 1.5 million fractures a year—mostly of the spine, hip, and wrist. The most common fracture occurs in the spine. When several spinal bones, or vertebrae, are fractured, the spinal column collapses, eventually resulting in a stooped posture known as kyphosis, or dowager's hump. Although hip fractures occur most often in women, one-quarter of all hip fractures occur in men. Health care costs for these fractures run about $14 billion a year and are expected to rise as the population ages.

FIGURE 3.5

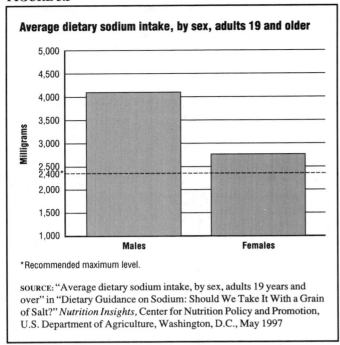

Average dietary sodium intake, by sex, adults 19 and older

*Recommended maximum level.

SOURCE: "Average dietary sodium intake, by sex, adults 19 years and over" in "Dietary Guidance on Sodium: Should We Take It With a Grain of Salt?" *Nutrition Insights,* Center for Nutrition Policy and Promotion, U.S. Department of Agriculture, Washington, D.C., May 1997

TABLE 3.15

Salt content, by food group

Food groups	Sodium, mg
Bread, cereal, rice, and pasta	
Cooked cereal, rice, pasta, unsalted, 1/2 cup	Trace
Ready-to-eat cereal,1 oz.	100-360
Bread, 1 slice	110-175
Popcorn, salted, 1 oz.	100-420
Pretzels, salted 1 oz	130-880
Vegetable	
Vegetables, fresh, or frozen, cooked without salt, 1/2 cup	Less that 70
Vegetables, canned or frozen with sauce, 1/2 cup	140-460
Tomato juice, canned, 3/4 cup	660
Vegetable soup, canned, 1 cup	820
Fruit	
Fruit, fresh, frozen, canned, 1/2 cup	Trace
Milk, yogurt, and cheese	
Milk, 1 cup	120
Yogurt, 8 oz.	160
Natural cheeses, 1-1/2 oz.	110-450
Process cheeses, 2 oz.	800
Meat, poultry, fish, dry beans, eggs, and nuts	
Fresh meat, poultry, fish, 3 oz.	Less than 90
Tuna, canned, water pack, 3 oz.	300
Bologna, 2 oz.	580
Ham, lean, roasted, 3 oz.	1,020
Peanuts, roatsed in oil, salted, 1 oz.	120
Other	
Salad dressing, 1 tsp.	75-220
Ketchup, mustard, steak sauce, 1 tbsp.	130-230
Soy sauce, 1 tbsp.	1,030
Salt, 1 tsp.	2,325
Dill pickle, 1 medium	930

SOURCE: "Where's the Salt?" in *Food Guide Pyramid Booklet 2000,* Center for Nutrition Policy and Promotion, U.S. Department of Agriculture, Washington, D.C., 2000

Preventing Osteoporosis

INCREASED CALCIUM INTAKE. Osteoporosis can be prevented. In 1997 the Institute of Medicine released the new Dietary Reference Intakes (DRIs) for calcium, established at levels compatible with the body's capacity to retain the most calcium. The recommendation for adolescents is 1,200 milligrams (mg). (See Table 3.6.) Apparently, calcium may enhance bone building in growing children and, starting at puberty, the body has a greater capacity to absorb and retain calcium.

Experts are especially concerned about growing girls, who generally have lower calcium intakes than boys. A U.S. Department of Agriculture (USDA) survey found that, while boys and young men ages 12 to 19 have average calcium intakes of 1,176 mg daily, girls and young women in the same age group consume just 777 mg of calcium per day. USDA studies have found that girls drink the least amount of fluid milk; tend to skip breakfast, depriving themselves of the calcium in cereals and milk; and consume the highest share of calories from fast foods, which have the lowest calcium contents, compared to foods prepared at home, schools, or restaurants.

Studies have also shown that the average American adult consumes just 500 to 700 mg of calcium daily, well below the new DRI of 1,000 mg. Postmenopausal women and older men also need to increase their calcium intakes. The DRI for those over 50 years old is 1,200 mg daily. (See Table 3.5.) As a person ages, his or her body becomes less efficient at absorbing calcium and other nutrients. Older adults also are more likely to have chronic medical problems and to use medications that may impair calcium

absorption. Moreover, inadequate vitamin D intake also calls for additional calcium intake. Major sources of calcium are cheese, milk, yogurt, tofu (made with calcium sulfate), broccoli, spinach, perch, and salmon.

VITAMIN D. Vitamin D helps prevent osteoporosis by assisting the body's absorption of calcium from the intestinal tract. More importantly, vitamin D helps maintain normal levels of calcium in the blood. By regulating the blood calcium levels, vitamin D helps make calcium available to bones for a process called mineralization. If the body has inadequate vitamin D, the bones are demineralized—they lose minerals to the blood in order to keep the calcium levels normal. Calcium is necessary for other body functions, including the contraction and relaxation of muscles (most notably the heart), nerve transmission, and blood clotting. If calcium is inadequate in the diet, it is withdrawn from the bones to maintain the levels of calcium in the blood and to regulate the heartbeat.

In recent years, experts have recognized that many elderly people get too little vitamin D. Skin conversion of vitamin D slows down with age. About 10 to 15 minutes of exposure to sunlight three times a week is generally enough for the body to synthesize its own vitamin D, but for older people, about 30 minutes of sun exposure is needed. Those who are housebound or who live in nursing homes are not likely to get enough sun. While milk is the primary source of vitamin D, older people tend to develop less tolerance for the lactose in milk. Furthermore, some may feel that milk is only for the young.

In 1997 new federal recommendations for vitamin D intake were issued. While the guidelines for adults up to age 50 remained at 200 International Units (IU), the Institute of Medicine set higher levels for those 51 to 70 years old (400 IU) and those over 70 (600 IU).

EXERCISE. Bones, like muscles, are living tissues, and they become stronger with exercise. Regular, weight-bearing exercise builds bone strength and prevents bone loss. It also helps prevent falls. People who exercise have a better sense of balance and better reflexes. They also build up more muscle padding to absorb the shock of a fall.

SODIUM

The mineral sodium makes up 40 percent of table salt, or sodium chloride, and plays an important role in regulating body fluids and blood pressure. Currently, there is no daily dietary requirement for sodium. Health authorities, including the American Heart Association and the National Academy of Sciences, recommend that sodium intake should be limited to no more than 2,400 milligrams (mg), about a teaspoon of salt, a day. The U.S. Department of Agriculture has found that Americans consume much more than the recommended limit, even when salt added at the table or during food preparation is not included. (See Figure 3.5). Table 3.15 shows the concentrations of sodium in the American diet.

A diet containing more than 2,400 mg of sodium is often associated with elevated blood pressure. Increased blood pressure can lead to hypertension, heart disease, stroke, and renal (kidney) disease. In the United States, nearly one in four people has hypertension, or high blood pressure. Clinical studies have shown that decreasing sodium intake lowers blood pressure in persons with or without hypertension. According to a study from the Northwestern University Medical School in Chicago, lowering lifetime salt intake by about one teaspoon a day would mean a 16 percent drop in coronary heart disease deaths and 23 percent fewer stroke deaths at age 55. Table 3.6 presents the Recommended Daily Intake for sodium.

CHAPTER 4

FOOD SPENDING

In 1999 (the latest year for which comprehensive Economic Research Service [ERS] data are available), Americans spent $691 billion for food. However, Americans do not spend their money today the way they did in the past. In the early years of the twentieth century, Americans spent about 40 percent of their income on food. According to the ERS of the U.S. Department of Agriculture (USDA), the share of disposable personal income Americans spent on food has declined steadily since 1970, although from 1992 to 1994 the percentage remained steady at about 11 percent. In 1999 the percentage of spending for food had fallen to 10.4 percent of disposable personal income. (Disposable personal income is the sum of personal consumption expenditures—spending on goods and services—plus savings and other miscellaneous expenditures).

Spending on food at home accounted for 6.2 percent of income; spending on food away from home, for 4.2 percent. (See Table 4.1.) Away-from-home meals and snacks accounted for 40 percent of the U.S. food dollar, up from 36 percent in 1970. Because the costs of restaurant meals include services (such as cooking the food, bringing it to your table, and washing dishes), as well as the cost of the food, the money spent does not purchase as much food as the money spent on food eaten at home. In addition, household food spending increased at a slower rate than household income during the 1990s. (See Table 4.2.)

DO AMERICANS SPEND MORE FOR FOOD THAN OTHERS?

In 1994 (the latest year for which comparable international data are available) Americans spent only 8.4 percent of their total personal consumption expenditures on food and alcoholic beverages consumed at home. (For international comparison, total personal consumption expenditures are used, instead of disposable personal income, because personal savings are seldom reported in the United Nations System of National Accounts, which furnished these data.) This compares with the 12.7 percent and 17.3 percent that Canada and the United Kingdom, respectively, spent on food and beverages. The average Japanese, with the greatest per person consumption expenditures ($21,830), spent almost 1 out of every 5 yen (17.6 percent) on food. (See Table 4.3.)

In 1994, in less-developed countries, food spending accounted for a much larger proportion of personal income. In India, Sri Lanka, and the Philippines, at-home food spending accounted for 50 percent or more of a household's budget. (See Table 4.3.)

In relation to total personal consumption budgets, Americans spend the least on food. The United States, with its varied climate and huge expanses of arable land, is not as dependent on imported food as most countries. Also, the farm-to-consumer distribution system is highly successful at moving large quantities of perishable food long distances with minimum spoilage. Finally, many American farmers have the most current information and use state-of-the-art farming tools in their work.

FOOD SPENDING IN AMERICAN HOUSEHOLDS

The *Consumer Expenditure Survey* (Bureau of Labor Statistics, Washington, D.C., 2000) found that while some expenditures, such as transportation, can vary significantly from year to year, food expenditures generally remain relatively stable. Average annual food expenditures rose 0.2 percent from 1997 to 1998 and 4.6 percent between 1998 and 1999. (See Table 4.4.)

Economists often describe food consumption as a relatively inelastic commodity. In other words, there is a limit to how much is spent on food. However, as income rises, the proportion spent on food declines, and more money is spent on personal services and discretionary spending. Expenditures for food require a large share of income when income is relatively low.

TABLE 4.1

Food expenditures by families and individuals as a share of disposable personal income, 1970–99

Year	Disposable personal income	Expenditures for food					
		At home[1]		Away from home[2]		Total[3]	
	Billion dollars	Billion dollars	Percent	Billion dollars	Percent	Billion dollars	Percent
1970	727.1	74.2	10.2	26.4	3.6	100.6	13.8
1971	790.2	78.1	9.9	28.1	3.6	106.2	13.4
1972	855.3	84.4	9.9	31.3	3.7	115.8	13.5
1973	965.0	93.1	9.7	34.9	3.6	128.0	13.3
1974	1,054.2	105.4	10.0	38.5	3.7	143.9	13.7
1975	1,159.2	115.2	9.9	45.9	4.0	161.1	13.9
1976	1,273.0	123.1	9.7	52.6	4.1	175.7	13.8
1977	1,401.4	131.8	9.4	58.5	4.2	190.3	13.6
1978	1,580.1	145.3	9.2	67.5	4.3	212.8	13.5
1979	1,769.5	162.2	9.2	76.9	4.3	239.1	13.5
1980	1,973.3	179.1	9.1	85.2	4.3	264.4	13.4
1981	2,200.2	191.0	8.7	95.8	4.4	286.8	13.0
1982	2,347.3	198.4	8.5	104.5	4.5	302.9	12.9
1983	2,522.4	209.0	8.3	113.7	4.5	322.7	12.8
1984	2,810.0	220.9	7.9	121.9	4.3	342.8	12.2
1985	3,002.0	230.7	7.7	128.6	4.3	359.3	12.0
1986	3,187.6	239.3	7.5	137.9	4.3	377.2	11.8
1987	3,363.1	249.0	7.4	146.3	4.3	395.3	11.8
1988	3,640.8	261.9	7.2	157.6	4.3	419.5	11.5
1989	3,894.5	280.9	7.2	165.5	4.3	446.4	11.5
1990	4,166.8	306.0	7.3	177.6	4.3	483.6	11.6
1991	4,343.7	319.5	7.4	183.1	4.2	502.6	11.6
1992	4,626.7	321.6	7.0	192.0	4.2	513.6	11.1
1993	4,829.3	327.7	6.8	204.9	4.2	532.6	11.0
1994	5,052.7	344.6	6.8	214.7	4.2	559.3	11.1
1995	5,355.7	360.4	6.7	222.6	4.2	583.1	10.9
1996	5,608.3	376.0	6.7	230.1	4.1	606.2	10.8
1997	5,885.2	390.3	6.6	239.1	4.1	629.4	10.7
1998	6286.2	395.5	6.3	263.8	4.2	659.3	10.5
1999	6639.7	410.5	6.2	280.9	4.2	691.3	10.4

[1] Food purchases from grocery stores and other retail outlets, including purchases with food stamps and WIC vouchers and food produced and consumed on farms (valued at farm prices) because the value of these foods is included in personal income. Excludes government-donated foods.
[2] Purchases of meals and snacks by families and individuals, and food furnished employees since it is included in personal income. Excludes food paid for by government and business, such as donated foods to schools, meals in prisons and other institutions, and expense-account meals.
[3] Total may not add due to rounding.

SOURCE: Economic Research Service, U.S. Department of Agriculture, Washington, D.C., 1997, 1999.

TABLE 4.2

Trends in household food spending, 1990–98

Item	1990	1995	1998	1990-98	1990-95	1995-98
	Dollars			Percent change		
U.S.average annual household income before taxes	33,152	37,255	42,584	28	12	14
Annual food spending per person	1,745	1,879	2,037	17	8	8
Food at home	1,025	1,198	1,211	18	17	1
Cereal and bakery products	153	191	187	22	25	-2
Meats,poultry,fish,and eggs	272	319	313	15	17	-2
Dairy	122	128	133	9	5	4
Fruits and vegetables	180	207	219	22	15	6
Sugar and sweets	38	49	51	34	29	4
Fats and oils	28	35	33	18	25	-6
Beverages	92	107	102	11	16	-5
Miscellaneous foods	139	162	174	25	17	7
Food away from home	720	681	826	15	-5	21

SOURCE: "Household Food Spending Rose More Slowly Than Income During the 1990's" in Noel Blisard, "Food Spending by U.S. Households Grew Steadily in the 1990's," *FoodReview*, Vol. 23, Issue 3, March 2001, Economic Research Service, U.S. Department of Agriculture, Washington, D.C.

The USDA Economic Research Services tracks the share of income Americans spend on food. Over the years 1960 to 1997, food eaten at home expenditures have decreased as a share of disposable income, while expenditures on food eaten away from home have remained constant. (See Figure 4.1.)

Not surprisingly, in 1999 the *Consumer Expenditure Survey* found that lower-income households spent less on food than did wealthier households. The poorest 20 percent of households spent an annual average of $2,715 on food, $1,834 (67 percent) of it at home. In contrast, the richest 20 percent spent a total of $8,568–$4,273 (50 percent) on food at home. (See Table 4.5.)

While richer families spent more on food than poorer families, they spent a smaller percentage of their income on food. The percentage of income before taxes spent on food varied from 33.7 percent for households with incomes of $5,000 to $9,999 to 7.7 percent for households with incomes of $70,000 and over. (See Table 4.6.)

DO THE POOR PAY MORE FOR FOOD?

In designing food-assistance programs, the federal government generally considers providing sufficient food dollars to enable low-income households to buy nutritious foods. For example, the monthly food stamp benefits consider the cost of the USDA's Thrifty Food Plan (TFP), "a market basket of suggested amounts of foods that make up a nutritious diet and can be purchased at a relatively low cost." These food prices are what the government knows poor households actually spend. Moreover, food stamp benefits are adjusted each year to allow for changes in the costs of these food items.

FIGURE 4.1

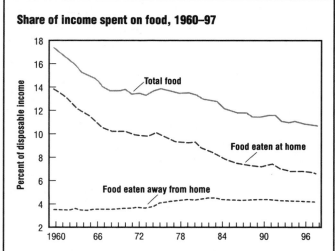

Share of income spent on food, 1960–97

SOURCE: Judith Jones Putnam and Jane E. Allshouse, "Figure 30: Share of income spent for food" in *Food Consumption, Prices and Expenditures, 1970–1997*, U.S. Department of Agriculture, Washington, D.C., 1998

TABLE 4.3

Percent of total personal consumption expenditures spent on food and alcoholic beverages to be consumed at home, by selected countries, 1994

Country	Percent of total personal consumption expenditures Food[2]	Percent of total personal consumption expenditures Alcoholic beverages	Personal consumption expenditures Total[3]	Personal consumption expenditures Food
	Percent	Percent	Dollars per person	Dollars per person
United States[1]				
ERS estimate	7.4	1.0	17,489	1,294
PCE estimate	8.4	1.7	17,489	1,469
Canada	10.3	2.4	11,581	1,193
United Kingdom	11.2	6.1	11,192	1,254
Netherlands	11.4	1.4	13,147	1,499
Hong Kong	12.3	0.7	12,602	1,550
Luxembourg (1991)	12.5	1.3	13,781	1,723
Singapore	13.8	1.6	9,268	1,279
Belgium	13.9	1.3	14,023	1,949
Sweden	14.6	2.7	12,217	1,784
Denmark	14.7	2.5	15,045	2,212
France	14.8	1.9	13,874	2,053
Australia	14.9	4.4	11,624	1,732
Austria	15.3	1.9	13,735	2,101
New Zealand	15.4[4]	NA	8,908	1,372
Finland	15.5	3.9	10,690	1,657
Puerto Rico	16.8	2.4	6,792	1,141
Italy	17.2	1.0	10,991	1,890
Germany	17.3[4]	NA	12,327	2,133
Japan	17.6[5]	NA	21,830	3,842
Spain (1993)	18.2	1.4	7,753	1,411
Ireland	19.0	12.0	8,157	1,550
Iceland	19.0	2.8	13,838	2,629
Norway (1993)	19.8	3.1	12,371	2,449
Israel	20.5	0.9	9,117	1,869
Portugal (1993)	23.2	3.1	5,238	3,557
Thailand	23.3	3.8	1,360	317
Switzerland	24.4[5]	NA	21,349	3,886
Fiji (1991)	24.4	3.6	1,352	918
Mexico	24.5	2.5	3,267	1,101
South Africa	27.5	6.5	1,846	508
Hungary	27.5	6.3	2,376	653
Cyprus	28.3	3.5	5,964	1,688
Korea, Republic of	29.1[5]	NA	4,596	1,544
Colombia (1992)	29.6	3.7	890	263
Peru (1990)	31.0[5]	NA	1,160	788
Greece	31.7	2.9	5,390	1,709
Malta (1993)	32.3	4.2	4,632	1,496
Ecuador (1993)	32.8	3.2	935	307
Bolivia	34.8[4]	NA	640	240
Venezuela	38.2[4]	NA	1,964	737
Sri Lanka	49.3	1.8	220	108
India	51.3	0.5	195	100
Philippines	55.6[4]	NA	659	364

NA = Not available.
[1]Two sets of figures are shown for the United States. The first set is based on estimates by the Economic Research Service (ERS) of the U.S. Department of Agriculture of U.S. food and beverage expenditures by families and individuals. The second set is based on the U.S. Department of Commerce estimates of personal consumption expenditures (PCE) for food and beverages, and is used by the UN. The ERS estimate is lower than the PCE estimate partly because it excludes pet food, ice, and prepared feed, which are included in the PCE estimates. The ERS estimates also deduct more from grocery store sales for nonfoods, such as drugs and household supplies, in arriving at the estimate for food purchases for at-home consumption.
[2]Includes nonalcoholic beverages.
[3]Consumer expenditures for goods and services.
[4]Food includes nonalcoholic and alcoholic beverages.
[5]Food includes nonalcoholic and alcoholic beverages and tobacco.

SOURCE: Judith Jones Putnam and Jane E. Allshouse, "Table 101 -- Percent of total personal consumption expenditures spent on food and alcoholic beverages that were consumed at home, by selected countries, 1994" in *Food Consumption, Prices and Expenditures, 1970–1997*, U.S. Department of Agriculture, Washington, D.C., 1998

TABLE 4.4

Annual expenditures of all consumer units and percent changes, 1997–99

Item	1997	1998	1999	Percent change 1997-98	Percent change 1998-99
Number of consumer units (000's)	105,576	107,182	108,465		
Income before taxes[1]	$39,926	$41,622	$43,951		
Average age of reference person	47.7	47.6	47.9		
Average number in consumer unit:					
Persons	2.5	2.5	2.5		
Earners	1.3	1.3	1.3		
Vehicles	2.0	2.0	1.9		
Percent homeowner	64	64	65		
Average annual expenditures	$34,819	$35,535	$37,027	2.1	4.2
Food	4,801	4,810	5,031	.2	4.6
At home	2,880	2,780	2,915	-3.5	4.9
Away from home	1,921	2,030	2,116	5.7	4.2
Housing	11,272	11,713	12,057	3.9	2.9
Apparel and services	1,729	1,674	1,743	-3.2	4.1
Transportation	6,457	6,616	7,011	2.5	6.0
Health care	1,841	1,903	1,959	3.4	2.9
Entertainment	1,813	1,746	1,891	-3.7	8.3
Personal insurance and pensions	3,223	3,381	3,436	4.9	1.6
Other expenditures	3,684	3,693	3,899	.2	5.6

[1]Income values are derived from complete income reporters only.

SOURCE: "Annual expenditures of all consumer units and percent changes, Consumer Expenditure Survey, 1997–99" in *Consumer Expenditures in 1999*, Bureau of Labor Statistics, U.S. Department of Labor, Washington, D.C., 2000

In *Do the Poor Pay More for Food?: Item Selection and Price Differences Affect Low-Income Household Food Costs* (Economic Research Service, Washington, D.C., November 1997), Phillip R. Kaufman, James M. MacDonald, Steve M. Lutz, and David M. Smallwood analyzed a number of studies to compare what low-income households and other households paid for the same food items. The researchers evaluated store surveys of food prices, household food expenditures surveys, and information from the *Census of Retail Trade*, the *Census of Population*, and USDA food stamp redemption.

According to Kaufman et al., some studies concluded that low-income households paid more for food items because they bought their foods in their neighborhoods, usually central cities or rural areas. Unlike suburban supermarkets, which generally offer lower prices, grocery stores in central cities and rural neighborhoods typically charge higher prices in order to cover higher business costs.

Buying in Central City and Rural Areas

The findings above suggest that low-income shoppers are less likely to visit supermarkets, where prices are usually lower. However, the researchers found that the use of various food outlets by low-income persons was similar to that of the rest of the population, and in fact, the percentage of food spending in supermarkets by low-income households was similar to that of the general population. (See Figure 4.2.) For example, the USDA reported that 76.7 percent of food stamps were redeemed in supermarkets and other large retailers (warehouse clubs and mass merchandisers), while *Census of Retailing* data showed that supermarkets and other large retailers accounted for 77.7 percent of national food sales.

Researchers found, however, that food spending in supermarkets varied by location within urban areas. In urban locations overall, supermarkets accounted for 74.6 percent of food stamp redemptions. However, within urban low-income neighborhoods, supermarkets accounted for only 64.3 percent of food stamp redemptions, and in low-income rural areas, supermarket food stamp redemptions were just half (52.8 percent) of all redemptions. (See Table 4.7.) The authors surmised that many low-income persons had no means to get to the supermarkets and might have had to pay more at smaller food stores. Table 4.8 illustrates weekly food costs for various food plans. For a family of four on the Thrifty Food Plan, weekly costs rose from $70.10 per week in 1990 to $86.20 per week in 1999, an increase of 23 percent.

Spending Less

Despite the fact that low-income households may face higher food prices, their spending patterns help them off-

TABLE 4.5

Consumer units and their average expenditures in 1999, by quintile

Item	All consumer units	Complete reporting of income — Total complete reporting	Lowest 20 percent	Second 20 percent	Third 20 percent	Fourth 20 percent	Highest 20 percent	Incomplete reporting of income
Number of consumer units (in thousands)	108,465	81,692	16,307	16,351	16,332	16,341	16,361	26,773
Lower limit	n.a.	n.a.	n.a.	$12,504	$24,184	$40,470	$66,476	n.a.
Consumer unit characteristics:								
Income before taxes[1]	$43,951	$43,951	$7,264	$18,033	$31,876	$52,331	$110,105	([1])
Income after taxes[1]	40,363	40,363	7,101	17,576	30,186	48,607	98,214	([1])
Age of reference person	47.9	47.9	51.6	51.6	46.5	44.1	45.9	47.8
Average number in consumer unit:								
Persons	2.5	2.5	1.8	2.2	2.5	2.8	3.1	2.6
Children under 18	.7	.7	.4	.6	.7	.8	.8	.7
Persons 65 and over	.3	.3	.4	.5	.3	.2	.1	.3
Earners	1.3	1.4	.7	.9	1.3	1.8	2.0	1.3
Vehicles	1.9	2.0	1.0	1.6	2.0	2.4	2.8	1.8
Average annual expenditures	$37,027	$39,174	$16,766	$24,850	$33,078	$46,015	$75,080	$30,820
Food	5,031	5,216	2,715	3,773	4,799	6,218	8,568	4,581
Food at home	2,915	3,010	1,834	2,472	2,832	3,637	4,273	2,683
Cereals and bakery products	448	461	292	372	424	555	661	418
Meats, poultry, fish, and eggs	749	758	504	655	713	911	1,008	726
Dairy products	322	338	199	267	319	411	492	285
Fruits and vegetables	500	515	318	436	487	589	744	462
Other food at home	$896	$938	$520	$742	$887	$1,171	$1,369	$793
Food away from home	2,116	2,206	882	1,301	1,968	2,580	4,295	1,897
Alcoholic beverages	318	348	161	224	280	385	687	245

[1]Components of income and taxes are derived from complete income reporters only.
[2]Value less than 0.5.
[3]No data reported.
[4]Data are likely to have large sampling errors.
n.a. Not applicable.

SOURCE: "Table 1. Quintiles of income before taxes: Average annual expenditures and characteristics, Consumer Expenditure Survey, 1999" in *Consumer Expenditures in 1999*, Bureau of Labor Statistics, U.S. Department of Labor, Washington, D.C., 2000

set these higher costs. Low-income households generally spend less than other households do for every food group, except fruit juices, vegetables, and eggs. Not surprisingly, they often choose more economical foods and lower-quality items. The researchers also found that low-income households tend to get more nutrients for their money, compared to foods bought by other households. They are more likely to buy unprocessed foods, such as beans and rice, and limit their purchases of convenience and prepared foods, which cost more money.

WHAT DID THE FOOD DOLLAR BUY IN 1999?

The money spent for food can be divided into the farm value (payment to farmers for the raw farm product) and the marketing bill. The marketing bill is the difference between the farm value of food produced on farms and the final cost to consumers at grocery stores and eating places. The marketing bill includes labor, packaging, transportation, depreciation, advertising, fuels and electricity, rent, taxes, and other expenses.

Consumers spent $618 billion on domestic farm foods in 1999. The estimated bill for marketing these foods was $498 billion or 80 percent of total spendings. The remaining $121 billion (20 percent) represents the farm value.

In 1999, of the total food bill, labor costs comprised the greatest expense (39 percent). In fact labor accounted for nearly half of all marketing costs. The farm value was the second largest piece—20 percent of the total. Packaging was the third largest component, accounting for 8 percent of food expenditures. (See Figure 4.3.)

TABLE 4.6

Consumer units and their average expenditures in 1999, by income before taxes

Item	Total complete reporting	Less than $5,000	$5,000 to $9,999	$10,000 to $14,999	$15,000 to $19,999	$20,000 to $29,999	$30,000 to $39,999	$40,000 to $49,999	$50,000 to $69,999	$70,000 and over
				Complete reporting of income						
Number of consumer units (in thousands)	81,692	3,909	7,588	8,639	6,995	11,560	9,453	7,381	10,999	15,168
Consumer unit characteristics:										
Income before taxes[1]	$43,951	$1,633	$7,631	$12,338	$17,311	$24,467	$34,353	$44,321	$58,473	$113,441
Income after taxes[1]	40,363	1,234	7,576	12,163	16,927	23,487	32,458	41,405	54,073	101,061
Age of reference person	47.9	39.1	55.3	55.8	50.9	48.8	45.8	44.7	43.9	45.8
Average annual expenditures	$39,174	$18,015	$14,926	$19,722	$24,366	$28,963	$35,077	$40,868	$49,615	$76,812
Food	5,216	2,873	2,576	2,917	3,821	4,322	5,060	5,823	6,527	8,725
Food at home	3,010	1,804	1,817	1,993	2,520	2,697	2,918	3,457	3,724	4,328
Cereals and bakery products	461	271	301	306	385	395	440	518	581	667
Cereals and cereal products	163	95	120	113	142	140	170	193	195	217
Bakery products	298	177	181	194	243	255	271	325	387	450
Meats, poultry, fish, and eggs	758	492	507	526	671	709	742	854	913	1,023
Beef	219	121	147	144	184	192	212	261	274	308
Pork	157	84	113	111	147	169	156	187	186	187
Other meats	99	70	60	81	90	101	94	104	124	125
Poultry	140	112	88	97	109	128	133	158	167	199
Fish and seafood	109	76	73	64	110	86	112	112	125	165
Eggs	33	28	25	29	32	32	36	33	36	39
Dairy products	338	204	190	220	266	296	334	383	428	499
Fresh milk and cream	128	93	79	90	109	113	140	137	162	170
Other dairy products	210	111	111	130	157	184	194	245	266	329
Fruits and vegetables	515	323	307	361	440	471	486	591	598	753
Fresh fruits	158	110	90	111	130	144	144	182	177	239
Fresh vegetables	153	90	93	107	131	141	149	172	176	224
Processed fruits	116	64	69	84	96	106	108	129	141	172
Processed vegetables	88	59	55	58	82	80	85	109	104	119
Other food at home	$938	$514	$510	$580	$758	$825	$916	$1,112	$1,204	$1,386
Sugar and other sweets	119	77	70	73	108	109	112	129	159	165
Fats and oils	85	56	52	55	86	82	88	107	95	107
Miscellaneous foods	438	212	225	261	340	378	431	532	567	668
Nonalcoholic beverages	254	143	150	173	205	226	250	289	333	354
Food prepared by consumer unit on out-of-town trips	43	26	14	19	18	30	36	56	50	91
Food away from home	2,206	1,069	759	923	1,301	1,625	2,142	2,365	2,803	4,398
Alcoholic beverages	348	271	100	180	205	267	292	345	443	696
Housing	12,315	6,403	5,735	7,112	8,319	9,423	10,862	12,644	14,873	23,066
Shelter	7,062	3,887	3,264	4,017	4,597	5,309	6,323	7,405	8,306	13,380
Owned dwellings	4,507	1,281	1,169	1,724	1,919	2,749	3,556	4,376	5,945	10,739
Mortgage interest and charges	2,517	585	359	482	712	1,207	1,958	2,680	3,631	6,546
Property taxes	1,080	382	430	634	650	770	851	930	1,311	2,324
Maintenance, repairs, insurance, other expenses	909	314	380	608	557	772	747	767	1,002	1,869
Rented dwellings	2,081	2,357	1,965	2,128	2,480	2,300	2,469	2,674	1,850	1,325
Other lodging	475	249	131	165	197	260	297	355	511	1,315
Utilities, fuels, and public services	2,368	1,311	1,505	1,825	1,944	2,159	2,297	2,491	2,795	3,411
Natural gas	262	129	162	199	233	232	241	270	302	398
Electricity	888	502	605	728	764	840	860	922	1,043	1,202
Fuel oil and other fuels	77	34	52	68	65	76	85	76	76	106
Telephone services	851	525	529	626	656	752	850	914	1,018	1,241
Water and other public services	290	120	157	204	226	258	261	309	356	463
Household operations	717	267	221	300	442	377	385	624	801	1,898
Personal services	357	113	102	104	260	164	178	353	441	933
Other household expenses	361	154	118	197	182	213	207	271	359	965
Housekeeping supplies	549	238	258	285	347	451	515	575	784	945
Apparel and services	1,871	993	699	893	1,356	1,553	1,904	1,677	2,139	3,625
Transportation	7,222	3,117	2,240	3,697	4,576	5,485	6,973	8,352	9,380	13,363
Health care	2,042	935	1,162	1,641	1,921	2,019	1,970	2,023	2,391	2,870
Entertainment	1,978	907	643	969	1,015	1,323	1,682	1,882	2,754	4,121
Personal care products and services	447	233	219	209	294	385	452	500	525	794
Reading	169	68	68	102	106	132	147	166	209	330
Education	593	863	354	267	255	309	347	425	602	1,430

TABLE 4.6

Consumer units and their average expenditures in 1999, by income before taxes [CONTINUED]

Item	Total complete reporting	Less than $5,000	$5,000 to $9,999	$10,000 to $14,999	$15,000 to $19,999	$20,000 to $29,999	$30,000 to $39,999	$40,000 to $49,999	$50,000 to $69,999	$70,000 and over
				Complete reporting of income						
Tobacco products and smoking supplies	315	259	223	257	295	305	336	376	391	328
Miscellaneous	959	391	355	381	580	742	890	986	1,107	2,004
Cash contributions	1,348	301	245	507	609	850	1,070	1,121	1,852	3,288
Personal insurance and pensions	4,352	401	306	590	1,014	1,849	3,092	4,548	6,421	12,17
Life and other personal insurance	408	139	119	168	169	264	342	349	517	970
Pensions and Social Security	3,944	262	187	423	844	1,585	2,750	4,199	5,904	11,202

[1] Components of income and taxes are derived from complete income reporters only
[2] Value less than 0.5.
[3] No data reported.
[4] Data are likely to have large sampling errors.

SOURCE: "Table 2. Income before taxes: Average annual expenditures and characteristics, Consumer Expenditure Survey, 1999" in *Consumer Expenditures in 1999,* Bureau of Labor Statistics, U.S. Department of Labor, Washington, D.C., 2000

FIGURE 4.2

Food shopping preferences, by income level, 1996

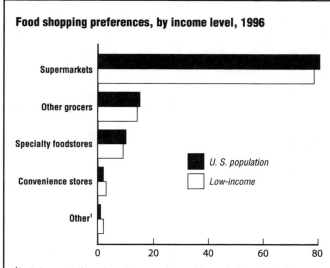

[1] Includes gas stations, drug stores, warehouse clubs, and other retail outlets.

SOURCE: Phillip R. Kaufman, James M. MacDonald, Steve M. Lutz, and David M. Smallwood, "Food shopping sources are similar among income levels" in *Do the Poor Pay More for Food?,* Economic Research Service, U.S. Department of Agriculture, Washington, D.C., 1997

TABLE 4.7

Food stamp redemptions by location and store type, 1996

Redemptions	Urban	Mixed	Rural	All areas
		Level of urbanization		
		Million dollars		
Total, all outlets	12,912	6,714	1,317	20,944
		Percent		
Share in supermarkets[1]	74.6	84.1	58.9	76.7
		Million dollars		
Total, low-income areas	5,594	2,507	543	7,128
		Percent		
Share in supermarkets[1]	64.3	79.9	52.8	66.3

[1] Supermarkets are defined as outlets authorized to offer food stamps and having $2 million or more in annual sales.

SOURCE: Phillip R. Kaufman, James M. MacDonald, Steve M. Lutz, and David M. Smallwood, "Food stamp redemptions by location and store type" in *Do the Poor Pay More for Food?,* Economic Research Service, U.S. Department of Agriculture, Washington, D.C., 1997

TABLE 4.8

Weekly food cost by type of family, 1990 and 1999

Assumes that food for all meals and snacks is purchased at the store and prepared at home.

Family type	December 1990				October 1999			
	Thrifty-plan	Low-cost plan	Moderate-cost plan	Liberal-plan	Thrifty-plan	Low-cost plan	Moderate-cost plan	Liberal-plan
Families								
Family of two:								
20–50 years	48.10	60.60	74.70	92.70	59.10	75.40	93.00	115.60
51 years and over	45.60	58.30	71.80	85.80	55.70	72.50	89.80	107.60
Family of four:								
Couple, 20–50 years and children—								
1–2 and 3–5 years	70.10	87.30	106.60	131.00	86.20	108.90	133.20	163.90
6–8 and 9–11 years	80.10	102.60	128.30	154.40	99.30	128.30	159.90	192.70
Individuals[1]								
Child:								
1–2 years	12.70	15.40	18.00	21.80	15.60	19.30	22.60	27.50
3–5 years	13.70	16.80	20.70	24.90	16.90	21.10	26.10	31.30
6–8 years	16.60	22.20	27.90	32.50	20.90	28.00	34.90	40.60
9–11 years	19.80	25.30	32.50	37.60	24.70	31.80	40.50	47.00
Male:								
12–14 years	20.60	28.60	35.70	42.00	25.60	35.80	44.50	52.20
15–19 years	21.40	29.60	36.80	42.60	26.30	36.90	46.00	53.00
20–50 years	22.90	29.30	36.60	44.30	28.20	36.60	45.60	55.20
51 years and over	20.90	27.90	34.30	41.10	25.50	34.80	42.90	51.50
Female:								
12–19 years	20.80	24.80	30.10	36.30	25.60	30.90	37.50	45.30
20–50 years	20.80	25.80	31.30	40.00	25.50	31.90	38.90	49.90
51 years and over	20.60	25.10	30.00	36.90	25.10	31.10	38.70	46.30

[1]The costs given are for individuals in four-person families. For individuals in other size families, the following adjustments are suggested: one-person, add 20 percent; two-person, add 10 percent; three-person, add 5 percent; five- or six-person, subtract 5 percent; seven-(or more) person, subtract 10 percent.

SOURCE: "No. 781. Weekly food cost by type of family: 1990 and 1999," *Statistical Abstract of the U.S.*, U.S. Census Bureau, 2000.

FIGURE 4.3

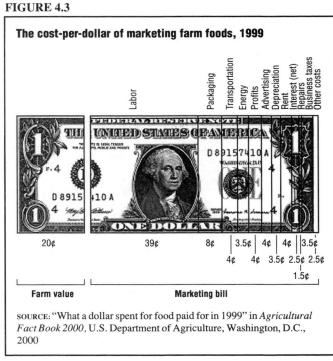

The cost-per-dollar of marketing farm foods, 1999

SOURCE: "What a dollar spent for food paid for in 1999" in *Agricultural Fact Book 2000*, U.S. Department of Agriculture, Washington, D.C., 2000

CHAPTER 5
SUPERMARKET SHOPPING

The Food Marketing Institute (FMI), an association of food retailers and wholesalers, annually surveys shopping behavior. One of their publications is *Trends in the United States—Consumer Attitudes and the Supermarket, 2000* (Washington, D.C., 2000). Although designed for food retailers, the survey reveals much about American food shopping habits.

SPENDING ON FOOD

Over the years spanning 1996 to 2000, family grocery spending has been fairly stable. In January 2000 the average weekly grocery bill was $85, down from $87 in 1999. Weekly grocery bills varied by the size and composition of the household. While a family of five or more spent an average of $130 per week on groceries, a household of one spent less than half that, at $49 per week. Households that earned less than $15,000 a year spent about $60 per week, while the wealthiest households, with incomes over $75,000, spent $123 a week. (See Table 5.1.)

Table 5.2 presents per-person weekly grocery expenses. Single-person households spent much more for their groceries ($49 on a per-person basis) than larger families ($23 per person in a family of five or more), which can take advantage of bulk buying. Men ($39 per week) spent more than women ($33), although women who worked less than 20 hours a week ($33) spent slightly less than women working 20 or more hours a week ($34). Single-person households and households without children ($40 per person) spent the most on weekly groceries. Shoppers across the country spent about the same weekly amount per person, although shoppers in the Midwest spent the least, $33 per week.

FREQUENCY OF SHOPPING AND USE OF STORE PRODUCTS AND SERVICES

In 2000 shoppers made an average of 2.2 trips per week to the supermarket. This has not changed much during the past 15 years.

The Food Marketing Institute (FMI) asked shoppers how often they used store products and services. Customers were most likely to participate in a frequent shopper program (67 percent) or buy private label or store brands (50 percent) at least once a week. About one-third used the fresh-food deli, in-store bakery, and self-check out/self-scanning services. (See Table 5.3.)

Over half of shoppers purchased natural or organic foods and gourmet, specialty, or ethnic foods at least once a month. Forty percent paid for their purchases with ATM or debit cards, and 27 percent paid for their groceries with credit cards. With the wide use of fax machines and the Internet, people are beginning to use these conveniences to order their groceries. Almost 1 in 12 (8 percent) of those surveyed reported ordering their groceries via the Internet. (See Table 5.3.)

EATING HOME-COOKED OR PREPARED MEALS

In 2000 most respondents surveyed by the FMI reported that they ate home-cooked meals at home either "pretty much every time" (34 percent) or "fairly often" (52 percent). When shoppers bought food that was prepared outside the home and taken home for consumption, 34 percent reported buying it at fast-food restaurants. An additional 22 percent bought take-out food from a restaurant, while 18 percent bought it in the supermarket. While supermarkets have held on to their share of the take-out food market over past years, fast-food establishments have seen a decline compared to 1996. (See Table 5.4.)

Supermarkets offer many timesaving products to make preparing meals at home easier. At least once a month, nearly two-thirds (62 percent) of shoppers bought pre-cut, cleaned, ready-to-cook vegetables, and 48 percent bought pre-cut, cleaned, and bagged salads. One-third bought frozen complete dinners at least once a month. One-quarter purchased precooked meat, poultry, and other main dishes at least once a month. (See Table 5.5.)

TABLE 5.1

Average weekly family grocery expenses by household size, income, region, and residence, 1996–2000

Question: About how much do you spend each week on groceries for your family? How much of this is spent at your primary grocery store?

	Jan. 2000 Base	Overall Total					Primary Store Total				
		Jan. 1996 $	Jan. 1997 $	Jan. 1998 $	Jan. 1999 $	Jan. 2000 $	Jan. 1996 $	Jan. 1997 $	Jan. 1998 $	Jan. 1999 $	Jan. 2000 $
Total	2,000	82	83	87	87	85	68	70	73	73	70
Size of Household											
One	364	47	48	51	51	49	40	41	43	44	42
Two	676	71	72	74	77	75	59	60	61	64	63
Three-four	655	93	97	100	102	101	77	81	84	87	82
Five or more	259	120	117	131	130	130	97	97	109	106	105
Income											
$15,000 or less	210	71	66	70	68	60	59	56	59	57	50
$15,001–$25,000	234	71	75	76	75	70	59	64	63	66	60
$25,001–$35,000	305	76	79	80	81	75	59	64	63	66	63
$35,001–$50,000	361	84	86	89	91	87	71	73	75	75	72
$50,001–$75,000	303	93	94	101	98	102	77	80	85	84	83
$75,001 or more	244	113	107	117	118	123	89	86	95	95	100
Region											
East	424	91	87	88	93	89	75	73	74	78	73
Midwest	526	77	77	86	83	77	63	66	72	70	64
South	610	80	84	87	83	85	67	71	73	70	71
West	440	83	85	89	92	91	67	70	73	76	73
Residence											
Urban	418	81	82	80	82	87	66	67	67	69	73
Surburban	517	87	90	95	95	92	71	75	79	79	75
Small town	590	82	79	83	87	82	67	68	69	72	68
Rural area	390	79	82	91	83	84	67	70	77	71	70

SOURCE: "Table 14: Average Weekly Family Grocery Expenses, 1996–2000, by Household Size, Income, Region and Residence," in *Trends in the United States: Consumer Attitudes & the Supermarket 2000,* Food Marketing Institute, Washington, D.C., 2000

TABLE 5.2

Average per person grocery expenses, 1996–2000

Question: About how much do you spend each week on groceries for your family? How much of this is spent at your primary grocery store?

	Jan. 2000 Base	Overall Total					Primary Store Total				
		Jan. 1996 $	Jan. 1997 $	Jan. 1998 $	Jan. 1999 $	Jan. 2000 $	Jan. 1996 $	Jan. 1997 $	Jan. 1998 $	Jan. 1999 $	Jan. 2000 $
Total	2,000	32	33	34	35	35	27	28	29	30	29
Gender											
Men	548	35	36	38	38	39	28	30	31	32	32
Women	1,452	31	32	33	35	33	26	27	28	30	28
Work 20+ hrs/wk	768	31	32	33	33	34	26	27	28	28	29
Work 0–19 hrs/wk	644	32	31	33	36	33	26	26	28	31	27
Type of Household											
With children	735	26	26	28	28	27	21	22	23	24	22
Aged 0–6	354	24	24	26	27	25	20	21	22	23	20
Aged 7–17	549	27	29	30	28	27	22	24	25	24	22
No children	1,209	38	38	39	41	40	32	33	33	35	34
Size of Household											
One	364	47	48	51	50	49	40	41	43	43	42
Two	676	35	36	37	38	38	29	30	31	32	31
Three-four	655	27	28	29	29	29	22	24	24	25	24
Five or more	259	22	21	24	23	23	18	18	20	20	19
Region											
East	424	34	34	35	37	36	29	29	29	33	29
Midwest	526	31	31	33	32	33	26	26	28	28	27
South	610	32	33	34	36	36	26	28	28	31	30
West	440	33	34	38	39	36	27	28	31	31	29

Calculated from average weekly grocery expenses and household size. Respondents who couldn't provide data were omitted from the calculation.

SOURCE: "Table 15: Average Per Person Grocery Expenses, 1996–2000," in *Trends in the United States: Consumer Attitudes & the Supermarket 2000,* Food Marketing Institute, Washington, D.C., 2000

TABLE 5.3

Shoppers' use of store products and services, 1996–2000

Question: Which of the following categories best describes how often you use/purchase (ITEM) at your primary grocery store?
(Base: Those who say their supermarkets have the product or service)

	Jan. 2000 Base	At Least Once a Month					Jan. 2000				
		Jan. 1996 %	Jan. 1997 %	Jan. 1998 %	Jan. 1999 %	Jan. 2000 %	At Least Once a Week %	1–3 Times a Month %	Less Than Once a Month %	Never %	Not Sure %
Frequent shopper program or savings club	450	70	81	84	85	88	67	21	3	8	*
Private label or store brands	927	88	86	86	84	85	50	35	10	4	1
Fresh food deli or delicatessen	847	75	76	77	72	73	33	40	14	12	*
In-store bakery	841	73	74	69	69	68	30	38	20	12	*
Self-checkout/self-scanning	142	x	x	x	63	63	35	28	8	26	2
Nutrition and health information for shoppers	666	58	58	63	63	57	27	30	21	20	1
Natural or organic foods	669	58	58	59	54	54	23	31	18	26	1
Gourmet, specialty or ethnic foods	659	47	53	53	54	52	16	36	20	27	*
Fresh seafood section	748	48	50	49	49	51	13	38	20	29	*
Gas pumps/gasoline	63	x	x	x	53	44	17	27	11	44	*
Juice bar	102	x	x	x	x	42	20	22	11	48	1
Accepts ATM or debit cards for purchases	823	35	39	37	42	40	20	20	10	51	*
In-store restaurant	289	x	32	30	21	28	9	19	24	48	1
Accepts credit cards for purchases	862	19	23	22	27	27	13	14	13	60	*
In-store pharmacy that fills prescriptions	502	28	28	25	26	23	3	20	19	57	*
In-store bank with a teller	416	30	33	36	24	21	11	10	12	66	*
Coffee bar that serves fresh, ready-to-drink coffees	354	32	33	36	24	21	11	10	12	66	*
Videos or movies for rent	335	36	32	29	24	20	7	13	16	64	*
Photo finishing department	517	21	27	20	20	18	*	18	32	50	*
Floral department	733	20	22	20	17	18	2	16	47	35	*
Dry cleaner	58	10	8	15	12	8	3	5	12	78	2
Online ordering	93	x	x	x	x	8	3	5	1	90	*
Home delivery	99	2	7	3	12	7	4	3	2	91	*
Child care	40	24	21	20	15	3	3	*	3	95	*

x = Not asked.
* = Less than 0.5 percent.
May not add to 100 percent due to rounding.

SOURCE: "Table 17, Shoppers' Use of Store Products and Services, 1996–2000," in *Trends in the United States: Consumer Attitudes & the Supermarket 2000,* Food Marketing Institute, Washington, D.C., 2000

In 2000 nearly one in five shoppers were more likely to buy prepared meals from a supermarket than from any other food establishment. People 65 and older (25 percent), low-income households (23 percent), and single-person households (23 percent) used supermarket takeout food most often. Women (19 percent) and unmarried persons (20 percent) were also more likely to use the supermarket as a source of meals eaten but not prepared at home. (See Table 5.6.)

Attitudes Toward Supermarket-Prepared Foods

In 1998 the FMI and *Prevention Magazine*, in *A Shopping for Health Report, 1998: Consumers' Interest in Nutritious Prepared Foods* (Washington, D.C., and Emmaus, PA, 1998), reported that most shoppers completely or mostly agreed that "prepared foods from the supermarket help me save time." While nearly 7 in 10 (69 percent) agreed that supermarket-prepared foods are more healthful than fast food, just 4 in 10 agreed that they are more healthful than packaged foods (43 percent of shoppers) or frozen foods (42 percent). (See Table 5.7.)

Over half (56 percent) of respondents indicated they were interested in the nutritional content of prepared foods from the supermarket. (See Table 5.7.) Shoppers who were most interested in nutritional information included working women (61 percent versus 47 percent of working men), college graduates (63 percent versus 52 percent of high school graduates and 47 percent of those who did not finish high school), and childless, married shoppers (62 percent versus 50 percent of childless singles).

CONCERN ABOUT NUTRITION

In 2000, 71 percent of consumers said they considered nutrition very important when they shopped for food, down from 78 percent in 1996. Taste, however, was rated the main concern by 89 percent of respondents. In 1994 nearly two-thirds (62 percent) of respondents indicated they were very concerned about the nutritional content of the food they ate. In 2000 under half (46 percent) said so.

Among various demographic groups, those who were most concerned about nutrition were people who live in the

TABLE 5.4

Sources of take-out food, 1996–2000

Question: Now I would like you to think about all meals that are eaten at home, but not prepared at home, are they purchased most often from a fast-food restaurant, a restaurant, a supermarket, convenience store, gourmet or specialty store, or from some other place? (Single answer accepted.)

	Jan. 1996 %	Jan. 1997 %	Jan. 1998 %	Jan. 1999 %	Jan. 2000 %
Base	1,001	1,018	1,002	1,002	1,000
Fast-food restaurant	48	41	37	31	34
Restaurant	25	21	20	21	22
Supermarket	12	22	20	20	18
Deli/pizza parlor/bagel shop coffee shop/donut shop	4	5	7	11	7
Gourmet or specialty store	3	7	4	5	5
Some other place	2	x	4	2	2
Convenience store	1	1	1	1	1
It varies (volunteered)	x	x	x	x	*
Friend's/relative's house	x	x	x	x	1
None	2	3	5	8	10
Don't know	2	x	2	1	2

Note: Modification to question wording in 2000.
x = Not asked/not mentioned.
* = Less than 0.5 percent.

SOURCE: "Table 34: Sources of Takeout Food, 1996–2000," in *Trends in the United States: Consumer Attitudes & the Supermarket 2000*, Food Marketing Institute, Washington, D.C., 2000

West (52 percent) and those in the highest income category (more than $75,000), with 59 percent. More than half of the people on medically restricted diets, as well as those who are vegetarians, were also very concerned about nutrition.

In 2000, among shoppers who were very or somewhat concerned about the nutritional content of their foods, 46 percent were concerned about the fat content of these foods, down 4 percentage points from the previous year. Concern about the fat content of food has sharply declined since its peak of 65 percent in 1995. In fact, concern for other nutritional factors, such as cholesterol, sodium, sugar, and calories, has also been decreasing. Although nutritionists stress that moderation and eating a balanced diet are the most important ways to achieve a healthy diet, only 2 percent and 6 percent of respondents respectively reported concern for "a balanced diet" and a desire to eat what is "good for us." (See Table 5.8.)

About 68 percent of those surveyed—an equal proportion of men and women—said their diets could be a lot or somewhat healthier. Only 8 percent felt their diet was as healthy as it could possibly be. Most (93 percent) shoppers claimed they were taking actions to ensure that their diet was healthy. Over two-thirds (68 percent) reported eating more fruits and vegetables. Nearly a quarter said they ate less fats and oils (23 percent) and less meat (22 percent). Other dietary initiatives reported included eating fewer snacks or junk foods and less sugar and salt. (See Table 5.9.)

TABLE 5.5

Supermarket products shoppers purchase for "meal solutions," 1997–2000

Question: How often do you buy the following items from (NAME OF PRIMARY GROCERY STORE)?

Base: 1,000 shoppers

	At Least Once a Month				Jan. 2000			
	Jan. 1997 %	Jan. 1998 %	Jan. 1999 %	Jan. 2000 %	At Least Once a Week %	1–3 Times a Month %	Less than Once a Month %	Never %
Frozen								
Frozen main dishes	40	38	40	37	11	26	21	41
Frozen side dishes	46	43	44	39	14	25	17	43
Frozen complete dinners	34	31	35	33	10	23	18	48
Value Added								
Pre-cut, cleaned and ready-to-cook vegetable items	57	67	67	62	34	28	14	24
Pre-cut, cleaned and bagged salads	45	50	50	48	19	29	19	32
Pre-cut, marinated or pre-seasoned meat or poultry that is ready to cook	32	31	33	26	8	18	16	56
Ready-to-eat, Ready-to-heat								
Pre-cooked meat poultry or other main dishes (chilled or hot)	33	29	34	26	7	19	22	50
Salad bar	21	22	22	16	5	11	11	65
Prepared ready-to-eat side dishes	28	28	30	26	7	19	22	52
Rotisserie or fried chicken	22	25	27	23	5	18	19	57
Sandwiches or pizza to go	24	28	27	21	6	15	17	60
Cooked-to-order hot foods for takeout	20	23	26	21	4	17	17	60
Hot food bar	21	20	22	17	4	13	16	62

May not add to 100 percent due to rounding.
Note: Modification of question wording in 2000.

SOURCE: "Table 37: Supermarket Products Shoppers Purchase for 'Meal Solutions,' 1997–2000," in *Trends in the United States: Consumer Attitudes & the Supermarket 2000*, Food Marketing Institute, Washington, D.C., 2000

Nutrition: A Key to Good Health

TABLE 5.6

Use of supermarket as a source of meals eaten at home but not prepared at home, 1996–2000

Question: Now I would like you to think about all meals that are eaten at home, but not prepared at home, are they purchased most often from a fast-food restaurant, a restaurant, a supermarket, convenience store, gourmet or specialty store, or from some other place? (Single answer accepted.)

	Jan. 2000 Base	Use Supermarket Most Often for Takeout Food				
		Jan. 1996 %	Jan. 1997 %	Jan. 1998 %	Jan. 1999 %	Jan. 2000 %
Total	1,000	12	22	20	20	18
Gender						
Men	286	13	28	23	24	14
Women	714	12	19	19	17	19
Work 20+ hrs/wk	377	8	18	18	15	19
Work 0–19 hrs/wk	320	17	21	19	20	19
Age						
15–24[1]	110	16	29	21	21	15
25–39	272	8	18	21	19	16
40–49	205	10	18	16	19	14
50–64	253	14	22	19	19	20
65 and older	155	25	32	26	21	25
Income						
$15,000 or less	106	18	24	22	30	23
$15,001–$25,000	125	12	21	29	20	14
$25,001–$35,000	154	14	23	22	19	19
$35,001–$50,000	189	12	19	19	15	20
$50,001–$75,000	144	10	18	17	19	11
$75,001 or more	119	5	21	14	16	13
Marital Status						
Married	577	12	19	19	17	16
Not married	397	14	25	22	24	20
Size of Household						
One	191	14	32	25	25	23
Two	337	15	22	19	18	16
Three–four	325	10	18	18	21	18
Five or more	127	10	18	20	9	15
Region						
East	209	x	22	16	19	17
Midwest	238	x	25	22	19	17
South	311	x	18	19	19	16
West	242	x	22	23	21	21

Note: Modification to question wording in 2000.
x = Not reported as a category in that year.
[1]Prior to 2000, the youngest age category was 18–24 years.

SOURCE: "Table 35: Use of Supermarket as a Source of Meals Eaten at Home But Not Prepared at Home, 1996–2000," in *Trends in the United States: Consumer Attitudes & the Supermarket 2000*, Food Marketing Institute, Washington, D.C., 2000

When shoppers were asked whether they had already taken steps to improve their diet because of nutritional concerns, the majority (79 percent) reported they had looked for and purchased low-fat food items, sought out low-cholesterol products (59 percent), and looked for and purchased products labeled as natural (59 percent). A third to a half reported making purchase decisions based on labeling information. About one-fifth of respondents said they were influenced by the "Five-a-Day" campaign to eat more fruits and vegetables (21 percent) and the "Food Guide Pyramid" (21 percent). (See Table 5.10.)

TABLE 5.7

Public opinion on prepared foods, 1998

Q: Please tell me if you completely agree, mostly agree, mostly disagree or completely disagree with each of the following statements about prepared foods from the supermarket.

	% who agree	
	1998	1997
Prepared foods from the supermarket help me save time.	85%	81%
Prepared foods from the supermarket are more healthful than food from fast-food restaurants.	69	65
I usually want to know the nutritional content of prepared foods from the supermarket.	56	N/A
Prepared foods from the supermarket are always fresh.	54	N/A
Prepared foods from the supermarket are more healthful than packaged foods I can buy off the shelf.	43	43
Prepared foods from the supermarket are more healthful than frozen foods.	42	38
Prepared foods from the supermarket help me eat healthfully.	36	36

SOURCE: "Attitudes Toward Prepared Food" in *A Shopping for Health Report, 1998: Consumer Interest in Nutritious Prepared Foods*, Food Marketing Institute and PREVENTION Magazine, Washington, D.C., and Erasmus, PA, 1998

TABLE 5.8

Nature of concern about nutritional content, 1996–2000

Question: What is it about the nutritional content of what you eat that concerns you most? What other concerns do you have? (Verbatim responses coded to categories listed below; multiple answers accepted.)
Base: 870 shoppers who are very or somewhat concerned about the nutritional content of the food they eat

	Jan. 1996 %	Jan. 1997 %	Jan. 1998 %	Jan. 1999 %	Jan. 2000 %
Fat content, low fat	60	56	59	50	46
Cholesterol levels	26	20	20	18	17
Food/nutritional value	6	11	12	17	12
Salt/sodium content, less salt	28	23	24	16	17
Sugar content/less sugar	12	11	12	9	13
Calories/low calorie	12	10	11	8	9
Chemical additives	7	6	6	8	7
Chemicals	3	1	*	x	x
Desire to be healthy/eat what's good for us	5	3	3	3	6
Preservatives	8	7	5	6	4
Vitamin/mineral content	12	5	x	2	3
Balanced diet	3	3	1	1	2
Carbohydrate content	1	1	2	1	2
Freshness/purity/no spoilage	5	4	4	3	3
Protein value	1	1	1	2	1
Fiber content	2	1	2	1	1
Nothing	1	1	1	3	3
Other	5	6	1	5	6
Don't know/no answer	4	4	3	4	7

x = Not reported as a category in that year.
* = Less than 0.5 percent.

SOURCE: "Table 41: Nature of Concern About Nutritional Content, 1996–2000," in *Trends in the United States: Consumer Attitudes & the Supermarket 2000*, Food Marketing Institute, Washington, D.C., 2000

TABLE 5.9

Changes for healthier diet, 1996–2000

Question: What, if anything, are you eating more of to ensure that your diet is healthy? What, if anything, are you eating less of to ensure that your diet is healthy? (Verbatim responses coded to categories listed below; multiple responses accepted.)

	Jan. 1996 %	Jan. 1997 %	Jan. 1998 %	Jan. 1999 %	Jan. 2000 %
Base	**1,007**	**1,011**	**1,000**	**1,004**	**1,000**
Any Dietary Change (NET)	97	93	90	95	93
More fruits/vegetables	77	78	78	71	68
More chicken/turkey/white meat	12	13	12	10	9
More fish	x	x	x	5	7
More low fat or skim milk products	x	x	x	5	5
More whole grains	x	x	x	4	4
More fiber	x	x	x	4	3
More juices	2	1	3	2	3
More protein	2	1	2	2	3
More starches (pasta, beans, rice)	6	3	3	4	2
More vitamin/mineral supplements/pills	2	2	2	2	2
More water/bottled water	*	2	3	2	2
More salads	x	x	x	x	2
More balanced diet/more variety	1	3	3	3	1
More fresh foods	3	2	2	2	1
More meat	x	x	x	1	1
More calcium	2	1	2	1	1
More organically grown/natural foods	1	1	*	1	1
More foods high in vitamins/minerals	1	1	1	*	1
More cereal	x	x	x	x	1
More dairy products	x	x	x	x	1
More bread/wheat	x	x	x	x	1
Less fats/oils	42	35	32	28	23
Less meats/red meats	32	35	33	27	22
Less junk food/snack food	18	24	25	22	18
Less sugar	20	16	18	14	17
Less salt/sodium/food low in salt/sodium	13	11	10	9	8
Less fried foods	x	x	x	6	7
Less dairy products	x	x	x	7	5
Less bread	2	1	5	3	3
Less cholesterol/food low in cholesterol	6	4	4	4	3
Less prepared/processed foods	3	3	4	1	3
Less soda	2	2	2	2	3
Less calories/food low in calories	1	1	1	1	1
Less carbohydrates	x	x	x	1	1

x = Not reported as a category in that year.
* = Less than 0.5 percent.

SOURCE: "Table 43: Changes for Healthier Diet, 1996–2000," in *Trends in the United States: Consumer Attitudes & the Supermarket 2000*, Food Marketing Institute, Washington, D.C., 2000

Nutrition: A Key to Good Health

TABLE 5.10

Actions consumers have taken due to nutrition concerns, 1996–2000

Question: The next series of questions focus on consumer issues related to grocery stores. I'd like to know if you personally have already done any of the following.
Base: 1,000 shoppers

	Have Already Done					Jan. 2000		
	Jan. 1996 Yes %	Jan. 1997 Yes %	Jan. 1998 Yes %	Jan. 1999 Yes %	Jan. 2000 Yes %	Yes %	No %	Don't Know %
Looked for and purchased products labeled as "low fat"	81	82	83	77	79	79	21	*
Looked for and purchased products labeled as "low cholesterol"	70	64	65	60	59	59	41	*
Looked for and purchased products labeled as "natural"	63	59	53	55	59	59	39	2
Started purchasing a product because of information on the product nutrition label	x	x	x	x	54	54	45	1
Looked for and purchased products labeled as "low salt"	61	57	56	53	52	52	48	*
Stopped purchasing a product because of information on the product nutrition label	x	x	x	x	46	46	53	2
Looked for and purchased products labeled as "organic"	40	37	35	33	37	37	61	2
Changed behaviors as a result of the safe handling labels on meat products	43	45	44	42	35	35	63	2
Changed purchases because someone in your household is on a medically restricted diet	33	35	33	32	31	31	69	*
Changed purchases because of the government's nutrition guidelines, also known as "Food Guide Pyramid"	23	27	27	25	21	21	78	2
Changed purchases because of the "Five-a-Day" campaign aimed at increasing purchases of fruits and vegetables	22	23	21	23	21	21	73	6
Changed purchases because someone in your household is a vegetarian or does not eat meat products	14	18	18	17	17	17	83	*

x = Not reported as a category in that year.
* = Less than 0.5 percent.
May not add to 100 due to rounding.
Note: Modification to question wording in 2000.

SOURCE: "Table 44: Actions Consumers Have Taken Due to Nutrition Concerns, 1996–2000," in *Trends in the United States: Consumer Attitudes & the Supermarket 2000*, Food Marketing Institute, Washington, D.C., 2000

CHAPTER 6
FOOD LABELING

HISTORY

In 1938 Congress enacted the Federal Food, Drug, and Cosmetic Act (52 Stat 1040) at a time when illnesses caused by nutritional deficiencies (for example, rickets, a bone disease caused by inadequate intake of vitamin D) were a common problem for the American people. The act required that the label of every processed, packaged food contain the name of the food, its net weight, and the name and address of the manufacturer or distributor. Certain products also had to carry a list of ingredients. The law further prohibited false or misleading statements in food labeling. In 1957, under the Poultry Products Inspection Act (PL 85-172), the U.S. Department of Agriculture (USDA) regulated the labeling of poultry products.

Although some scientific evidence pointed to the possible link between blood cholesterol and heart disease during the 1950s, it was not until 1965 that the Food and Drug Administration (FDA) permitted fat and cholesterol statements on food labels. Products could carry the statement saying, "Information on fat and cholesterol is provided for individuals who, on the advice of a physician, are modifying their dietary intake of fat and cholesterol."

In 1969 the White House Conference on Food, Nutrition, and Health studied the American diet to determine deficiencies. The Conference recommended that the federal government establish a system for providing nutrient content information on food labels to promote public awareness of proper nutrition. Consequently, in 1973, the FDA for the first time ordered fortified foods (foods with one or more added nutrients) and those making a health claim to carry nutrition labeling. For all other food products, nutrition labeling was voluntary. Manufacturers that provided nutrient content information on their food labels were required to list the calorie content as well as the grams of protein, carbohydrate, and fat in a single serving of food. The FDA also required a list of seven vitamins and minerals. See Table 6.1 for a sample FDA nutrition label.

TABLE 6.1

Sample Food and Drug Administration nutrition label

Nutrition Information	Per Serving	Percentage of U.S. Recommended Daily Allowances (U.S. RDA)	
Serving size	5oz.	Protein	10
Servings per container	4	Vitamin A	*
Calories	250	Vitamin C	*
Protein	9g	Thiamine	8
Carbohydrate	19g	Riboflavin	5
Fat	11g	Niacin	2
		Calcium	20
		Iron	4

*Contains less than 2% of the U.S. RDA of this nutrient

SOURCE: U.S. Food and Drug Administration, Washington, D.C.

In the late 1970s nutritionists and other experts who recognized the relationship between dietary practices and long-term health pushed for food labeling reforms. In 1980, in response to the public's desire for authoritative, consistent guidelines on diet and health, the USDA and the Department of Health and Human Services (HHS) first published *Nutrition and Your Health: Dietary Guidelines for Americans.* (Washington, D.C.)

In 1984 the FDA added sodium to the list of required nutrients on food labels. The addition of potassium to the nutrient list was optional. The following year, the agency allowed such terms as "low sodium" to be added as nutrient claims.

The federal government formally acknowledged the role of diet in such major chronic diseases as heart disease and cancer in the 1988 *Surgeon General's Report on Nutrition and Health.* The 1989 National Research Council report, *Diet and Health: Implications for Reducing Chronic Disease* (Washington, D.C.) offered scientific evidence of the growing acceptance of this relationship.

FIGURE 6.1

How to read a nutrition facts label

Macaroni & cheese

Nutrition Facts
Serving Size 1 cup (228g)
Servings Per Container 2

Amount Per Serving

Calories 250	Calories from Fat 110

% Daily Value*

Total Fat 12g	**18%**
Saturated Fat 3g	**15%**
Cholesterol 30mg	**0%**
Sodium 470mg	**20%**
Total Carbohydrate 31g	**10%**
Dietary Fiber 0g	**0%**
Sugars 5g	
Protein 5g	

Vitamin A	4%
Vitamin C	2%
Calcium	20%
Iron	4%

* Percent Daily Values are based on a 2,000 calorie diet. Your daily values may be higher or lower depending on your calorie needs:

		Calories:	2,000	2,500
Total Fat	Less than		65g	80g
Sat Fat	Less than		20g	25g
Cholesterol	Less than		300mg	300mg
Sodium	Less than		2,400mg	2,400mg
Total Carbohydrate			300g	375g
Dietary Fiber			25g	30g

Quick guide to % daily value

5% or less is low
20% or more is high

Start here →

Limit these nutrients

Get enough of these nutrients

Footnote

SOURCE: "How to Read a Nutrition Facts Label" in *Dietary Guidelines for Americans, 2000*, U.S. Department of Agriculture, Washington, D.C., 2000

TABLE 6.2

The nutritional information panel

UNDER THE LABEL'S "NUTRITION FACTS" PANEL, MANUFACTURERS ARE REQUIRED TO PROVIDE INFORMATION ON CERTAIN NUTRIENTS. THE MANDATORY (UNDERLINED) AND VOLUNTARY COMPONENTS AND THE ORDER IN WHICH THEY MUST APPEAR ARE:

- total calories
- calories from fat
- calories from saturated fat
- total fat
- saturated fat
- polyunsaturated fat
- monounsaturated fat
- cholesterol
- sodium
- potassoium
- total carbohydrate
- dietary fiber
- souble fiber
- insoluble fiber
- sugars
- sugar alcohol (for example, the sugar substitutes xylitol, mannitol and sorbitol)
- other carbohydrate (the difference between total carbohydrate and the sum of dietary fiber, sugars, and sugar alcohol if declared)
- protein
- vitamin A
- percent of vitamin A present as beta–carotene
- vitamin C
- calcium
- iron
- other essential vitamins and minerals

SOURCE: "Nutritional information panel" in *The New Food Label,* U.S. Food and Drug Administration, Washington, D.C., 1999

ure 6.1.) Manufacturers who wish to present nutrition labeling in a second language may do so either on a separate label or on the same label.

The FDA requires that the following nutrients must be listed in order on the food label: total calories, calories from fat, total fat, saturated fat, cholesterol, sodium, total carbohydrate, dietary fiber, sugars, protein, vitamin A, vitamin C, calcium, and iron. In addition, manufacturers may choose to include several additional nutrients. (See Table 6.2.) If the food manufacturer makes a claim about an optional component, or if the food is fortified or enriched, the relevant nutrition information for these components becomes mandatory.

The FDA selects nutrients for listing based on current health concerns, and the order they must be listed in reflects their importance. Such nutrients as thiamine, riboflavin, and niacin are no longer required on the label because deficiencies of these B vitamins are no longer considered public health problems.

Serving Sizes

With the passage of the NLEA, the FDA requires that a serving size reflect the amount of food a person actually eats at one time. This is determined primarily by nutritional food consumption surveys. Serving sizes must be stated in terms of both household and metric measurements.

In 1990 Congress passed the Nutrition Labeling and Education Act (NLEA; PL 101-535), authorizing the FDA to require all packaged foods to carry nutrition labeling. The NLEA is intended to provide consumers with uniform and accurate nutrition information about the foods they eat.

Although under no congressional mandate, the Food Safety and Inspection Service (FSIS) of the USDA has coordinated efforts with the FDA by requiring meat and poultry labeling. While the FSIS is responsible for nutrition labels on raw meat and poultry products, the FDA is responsible for food labels on all other food products. Final implementation of the new rules became effective in 1994.

THE NUTRITION LABEL

Previously referred to as "Nutrition Information per Serving," the nutrition label is now called "Nutrition Facts." The new label provides more complete, useful, and accurate nutrition information than before. (See Fig-

Percent of Daily Value

A dietary reference term called "Percent Daily Value" shows how a food fits into a person's daily diet. According to the FDA, consumers should keep in mind that the listed Daily Value is not a recommended intake of a particular nutrient. Rather, the Percent Daily Value enables the consumer to see what proportion of the Daily Value for each nutrient a serving of a particular food offers. (See Figure 6.1.)

For example, a food label may state that a certain food contains 5 grams of saturated fat per serving. The current health recommendation for daily saturated fat is 20 grams or less. Although 5 grams of saturated fat may seem like a small amount, the Percent Daily Value shows that 5 grams of fat actually constitute 25 percent of the total Daily Value for saturated fat.

Food labels also allow for comparisons between foods. Figure 6.2 presents labels for two food items, reduced fat milk and chocolate nonfat milk. The reduced

FIGURE 6.2

A comparison of reduced and nonfat milk

SOURCE: "Comparison Example #2" in *Guidance on How to Understand and Use the Nutrition Facts Panel on Food Labels,* Center for Food Safety and Applied Nutrition, U.S. Food and Drug Administration, June 2000

TABLE 6.3

Daily reference values recommended by the U.S. Food and Drug Administration*

Food Component	DRV
fat	65 grams (g)
saturated fatty acids	20 g
cholesterol	300 milligrams (mg)
total carbohydrate	300 g
fiber	25 g
sodium	2,400 mg
potassium	3,500 mg
protein**	50 g

*Based on 2,000 calories a day for adults and children over 4 only
**DRV for protein does not apply to certain populations; Reference Daily Intake (RDI) for protein has been established for these groups: children 1 to 4 years: 16 g; infants under 1 year: 14 g; pregnant women: 60 g; nursing mothers: 65 g.

SOURCE: U.S. Food and Drug Administration, Washington, D.C., 2001

TABLE 6.4

Recommended energy intake by age, sex, and activity level

Category	Age	Light Activity	Moderate Activity	Heavy Activity
Children	4-6		1,800	
	7-10		2,000	
Males	11-14		2,500	
	15-18		3,000	
	19-24	2,700	3,000	3,600
	25-50	3,000	3,200	4,000
	51+		2,300*	
Females	11-18		2,200	
	19-24	2,000	2,100	2,600
	25-50	2,200	2,300	2,800
	51+		1,900*	

Pregnant women in their second and third trimesters should add 300 calories to the figure the table indicates for their age.
Nursing mothers should add 500.
* based on light to moderate activity

Activity Levels
Very Light: Driving, typing, painting, laboratory work, ironing, sewing, cooking, playing cards, playing a musical instrument, other seated or standing activities
Light: Housecleaning, child care, garage work, electrical trade work, carpentry, restaurant work, golf, sailing, table tennis, walking on a level surface at 2.5 to 3 miles per hour
Moderate: Weeding, hoeing, carrying a load, cycling, skiing, tennis, dancing, walking 3.5 to 4 miles per hour
Heavy: Heavy manual digging, tree felling, basketball, climbing, football, soccer, carrying a load uphill

SOURCE: "Recommended Energy Intake" in "Recommended Daily Allowances," National Academy of Sciences, Washington, D.C.

TABLE 6.5

Reference daily intakes (RDIs) for vitamins and nutrients

Nutrient	Amount
vitamin A	5,000 International Units (IU)
vitamin C	60 milligrams (mg)
thiamin	1.5 mg
riboflavin	1.7 mg
niacin	20 mg
calcium	1.0 gram (g)
iron	18 mg
vitamin D	400 IU
vitamin E	30 IU
vitamin B6	2.0 mg
folic acid	0.4 mg
vitamin B12	6 micrograms (mcg)
phosphorus	1.0 g
iodine	150 mcg
magnesium	400 mg
zinc	15 mg
copper	2 mg
biotin	0.3 mg
pantothenic acid	10 mg

Based on National Academy of Sciences' 1968 Recommended Dietary Allowances.

SOURCE: U.S. Food and Drug Administration, Washington, D.C., 2001

FIGURE 6.3

Fruit dessert for children less than two years old

Nutrition Facts
Serving Size 1 jar (140g)

Amount Per Serving

Calories 110

Total Fat	0g
Sodium	10mg
Total Carbohydrate	27mg
Dietary Fiber	4g
Sugars	0g
Protein	0g

% Daily Value

Protein 0%	•	Vitamin A 6%
Vitamin C 45%	•	Calcium 2%
Iron 2%		

SOURCE: *A Food Labeling Guide,* U.S. Food and Drug Administration, Washington, D.C., 1999

fat milk contains 15 percent of the Daily Value for saturated fat and 8 percent of the total fat Daily Value, compared to the nonfat milk's zero. Both provide the same percent Daily Values for total carbohydrate, protein, calcium, and the vitamins listed. The reduced fat milk contains 50 percent more calories than the nonfat milk.

Daily Values (DVs) are derived from two sets of dietary standards—*Daily Reference Values* (DRVs) and *Reference Daily Intakes* (RDIs). Although these two dietary references serve as the basis for calculating daily values, only the DV term is used for food labeling.

DRVs are dietary references for macronutrients that are sources of energy (fat, saturated fat, protein, and total carbohydrates, including fiber) and for cholesterol, sodium, and potassium that do not contribute calories. (See Table 6.3.) DRVs for the energy sources are based on the number of calories consumed each day.

For the purpose of food labeling, the FDA and the USDA base the DRVs and, consequently, the Percent Daily Values on a 2,000-calorie-a-day diet. The number of calories a person needs is based on body size, age, height, weight, activity level, and metabolism. The National Academy of Sciences has prepared recommendations for daily caloric intake based on these factors. (See Table 6.4.) Although many consumers require more than 2,000 calories a day, health experts agree that 2,000 calories represent the caloric requirement for postmenopausal women—the group with the highest risk for excessive intake of calories and fat. However, manufacturers may include Daily Values for other calorie levels if they so desire. Many food packages include Daily Values for a 2,500-calorie diet. (See Figure 6.1.)

Regardless of a person's recommended calorie intake, the DRVs are calculated as follows:

• Fat: no more than 30 percent of calories.

• Saturated fat: no more than 10 percent of calories.

• Carbohydrate: no more than 60 percent of calories.

• Fiber: no more than 11.5 grams (g) of fiber per 1,000 calories.

• Protein: no more than 10 percent of calories. (The DRV for protein applies only to adults and children over age four. RDIs for protein have been established for other groups—children ages one to four, 14 g; pregnant women, 60 g; and nursing mothers, 65 g.)

Let's assume, for example, that a person's daily caloric intake is 2,000. The recommended DRV for saturated fat is no more than 10 percent of the total daily caloric intake. The person should, therefore, limit his or her calories from saturated fat to 200. A gram of fat has 9 calories, which means that the person should consume no more than 22 grams of saturated fat.

Based on scientific evidence that links certain nutrients and diseases, the federal government has established DRV parameters for these nutrients:

• Total fat—less than 65 g.

• Saturated fat—less than 20 g.

- Cholesterol—less than 300 milligrams (mg.)
- Sodium—less than 2,400 mg.

Pursuant to the NLEA, the *Reference Daily Intakes* (RDIs, Table 6.5) replaced the term U.S. RDAs (U.S. Recommended Daily Allowances), which was introduced in 1973 by the FDA as a label reference value for vitamins, minerals, and protein in voluntary nutrition labeling. The RDIs are also used in calculating the Daily Values for food labels.

Nutrition Labeling for Children's Food

Food labels for children under two years of age cannot carry information on calories from fat and saturated fat. In addition, labels cannot have quantitative amounts for saturated fat, polyunsaturated fat, monounsaturated fat, and cholesterol. (See Figure 6.3.) This is to prevent parents from thinking that infants and toddlers should limit their fat intake when, in fact, fat is necessary for healthy growth and development at this stage of life. Food labels for children ages two to four cannot include Percent Daily Values for macronutrients such as carbohydrates and fiber because the FDA has not determined Daily Values for this age group. (See Figure 6.4.)

NUTRIENT CONTENT CLAIMS IN FOOD LABELS

The NLEA also specifies what terms may be used to describe the level of a nutrient in a food and how the terms can be used. The NLEA permits 11 basic terms. Table 6.6 explains the criteria for the following nutrient content claims:

- Free
- Low
- Very Low
- Percent fat free
- Substantially less
- No added sugars
- Without added sugars
- Reduced/less
- Light
- Fewer

The term "free" means that a product contains no amount of, or only trivial or "physiologically inconsequential" amounts of, the nutrient. "Low" can be used on foods that can be eaten frequently without exceeding the Daily Value for that nutrient. (See Table 6.6 for synonyms for the terms "free" and "low.")

Manufacturers are allowed to use alternative spellings of these terms and their synonyms—for example, lite (light) or lo (low)—as long as the alternative word is not misleading.

FIGURE 6.4

Fruit dessert for children aged two years to four years

Nutrition Facts
Serving Size 1 jar (140g)

Amount Per Serving

Calories 110	Calories from Fat 0
Total Fat	0g
Saturated Fat	0g
Cholesterol	0mg
Sodium	10mg
Total Carbohydrate	27mg
Dietary Fiber	4g
Sugars	0g
Protein	0g

% Daily Value

Protein 0%	•	Vitamin A 6%
Vitamin C 45%	•	Calcium 2%
Iron 2%		

SOURCE: *A Food Labeling Guide*, U.S. Food and Drug Administration, Washington, D.C., 1999

Nutritionally Altered Products

The NLEA allows manufacturers to compare nutritionally altered products with regular products (referred to as reference foods) by making a relative claim, using such terms as reduced, less, light, fewer, and more. The regular product may be an individual food or a group of foods representative of the type of food. A relative claim must include the percent difference and the identity of the regular food.

The term "reduced" means that a nutritionally altered product contains at least 25 percent less of a nutrient or of calories than the reference food. The terms "less" or "fewer" mean that a food, whether altered or not, contains 25 percent less of a nutrient or of calories than the reference food.

The term "light" or "lite" can be used to describe either of two things:

- A nutritionally altered product that contains one-third fewer calories or half the fat of the reference food. If the food derives 50 percent or more of its calories from fat, the reduction must be 50 percent of the fat.

- A low-calorie, low-fat food in which the sodium content has been reduced by 50 percent. The description "light in sodium" may be used if the food has at least 50 percent less sodium than a reference food.

TABLE 6.6

U.S. Food and Drug Administration definitions for nutrient content claims

Nutrient	Free	Low	Reduced/Less	Comments
	Synonyms for "Free" : "Zero", "No", "Without", "Trivial Source of", "Negligible Source of", "Dietarily Insignificant Source of". Definitions for "Free" for meals and main dishes are the stated values per labeled serving.	Synonyms for "Low": "Little", ("Few" for Calories), "Contains a Small Amount of", "Low Source of".	Synonyms for "Reduced/Less": "Lower" ("Fewer" for Calories). "Modified" may be used in statement of identity. Definitions for meals and main dishes are same as for individual foods on a per 100 g basis.	For "Free", "Very Low", or "Low", must indicate if food meets a definition without benefit of special processing, alteration, formulation or reformulation; e.g., "broccoli, a fat-free food" or "celery, a low calorie food".
Calories 21 CFR 101.60(b)	Less than 5 cal per reference amount and per labeled serving.	40 cal or less per reference amount (and per 50 g if reference amount is small). Meals and main dishes: 120 cal or less per 100 g.	At least 25% fewer calories per reference amount than an appropriate reference food. Reference food may not be "Low Calorie". Uses term "Fewer" rather than "Less".	"Light" or "Lite": If 50% or more of the calories are from fat, fat must be reduced by at least 50% per reference amount. If less than 50% of calories are from fat, fat must be reduced at least 50% or calories reduced at least 1/3 per reference amount. "Light" or "Lite" meal or main dish product meets definition for "Low Calorie" or "Low Fat" meal and is labeled to indicate which definition is met. For dietary supplements: Calorie claims can only be made when the reference product is greater than 40 calories per serving.
Total Fat 21 CFR 101.62(b)	Less than 0.5 g per reference amount and per labeled serving (or for meals and main dishes, less than 0.5 g per labeled serving). Not defined for meals or main dishes.	3 g or less per reference amount (and per 50 g if reference amount is small). Meals and main dishes: 3 g or less per 100 g and not more than 30% of calories from fat.	At least 25% less saturated fat per reference amount than an appropriate reference food. Reference food may not be "Low Fat".	"__% Fat Free": OK if meets the requirements for "Low Fat". 100% Fat Free: Food must be "Fat Free". "Light"—see above. For dietary supplements: Calorie claims cannot be made for products that are 40 calories or less per serving.
Saturated Fat 21 CFR 101.62(c)	Less than 0.5 g saturated fat and less than 0.5 g trans fatty acids per reference amount and per labeled serving (or for meals and main dishes, less than 0.5 g saturated fat and less than 0.5 g trans fatty acids per labeled serving). No ingredient that is understood to contain saturated fat except as noted below(*).	1 g or less per reference amount and 15% or less of calories from saturated fat. Meals and main dishes: 1 g or less per 100 g and less than 10% of calories from saturated fat.	At least 25% less saturated fat per reference amount than an appropriate reference food. Reference food may not be "Low Saturated Fat".	Next to all saturated fat claims, must declare the amount of cholesterol if 2 mg or more per reference amount; and the amount of total fat if more than 3 g per reference amount (or 0.5 g or more of total fat for "Saturated Fat Free"). For dietary supplements: saturated fat claims cannot be made for products that are 40 calories or less per serving.
Cholesterol 21 CFR 101.62(d)	Less than 2 mg per reference amount and per labeled serving (or for meals and main dishes, less than 2 mg per labeled serving). No ingredient that contains cholesterol except as noted below(*). If less than 2 mg per reference amount by special processing and total fat exceeds 13 g per reference amount and labeled serving, the amount of cholesterol must be "Substantially Less" (25%) than in a reference food with significant market share (5% of market).	20 mg or less per reference amount (and per 50 g of food if reference amount is small). If qualifies by special processing and total fat exceeds 13 g per reference and labeled serving, the amount of cholesterol must be "Substantially Less" (25%) than in a reference food with significant market share (5% of market). Meals and main dishes: 20 mg or less per 100 g.	At least 25% less cholesterol per reference amount than an appropriate reference food. Reference food may not be "Low Cholesterol".	Cholesterol claims only allowed when food contains 2 g or less saturated fat per reference amount; or for meals and main dish products—per labeled serving size for "Free" claims or per 100 g for "Low" and "Reduced/Less" claims. Must declare the amount of total fat next to cholesterol claim when fat exceeds 13 g per reference amount and labeled serving (or per 50 g of food if reference amount is small), or when the fat exceeds 19.5 g per labeled serving for main dishes or 26 g for meal products. For dietary supplements: Cholesterol claims cannot be made for products that are 40 calories or less per serving.
Sodium 21 CFR 101.61	Less than 5 mg per reference amount and per labeled serving (or for meals and main dishes, less than 5 mg per labeled serving). No ingredient that is sodium chloride or generally understood to contain sodium except as noted below(*).	140 mg or less per reference amount (and per 50 g if reference amount is small). Meals and main dishes: 140 mg or less per 100 g.	At least 25% less sodium per reference amount than an appropriate reference food. Reference food may not be "Low Sodium".	"Light" (for sodium reduced products): If food is "Low Calorie" and "Low Fat" and sodium is reduced by at least 50%. "Light in Sodium": If sodium is reduced by at least 50% per reference amount. Entire term "Light in Sodium" must be used in same type, size, color & prominence. "Light in Sodium" for meals = "Low in Sodium".

In addition, the term "light" can be used to describe such properties as color and texture, as long as the label explains the intended use of the term—for example, "light brown sugar" and "light and fluffy."

A serving of food bearing the "more" claim must contain at least 10 percent more of the Daily Value for the particular nutrient than a similar reference food. The 10 percent of Daily Value also applies to such

TABLE 6.6

U.S. Food and Drug Administration definitions for nutrient content claims

Nutrient	Free	Low	Reduced/Less	Comments
				"Very Low Sodium": 35 mg or less per reference amount (and per 50 g if reference amount is small). For meals and main dishes: 35 mg or less per 100 g. "Salt Free" must meet criterion for "Sodium Free". "No Salt Added" and "Unsalted" must note conditions of use and must declare "This is Not A Sodium Free Food" on information panel if food is not "Sodium Free". "Lightly Salted": 50% less sodium than normally added to reference food and if not "Low Sodium", so labeled on information panel.
Sugars 21 CFR 101.60(c)	"Sugar Free": Less than 0.5 g sugars per reference amount and per labeled serving (or for meals and main dishes, less than 0.5 g per labeled serving). No ingredient that is a sugar or generally understood to contain sugars except as noted below(*). Disclose calorie profile (e.g., "Low Calorie").	Not Defined. No basis for recommended intake.	At least 25% less sugars per reference amount than an appropriate reference food. May not use this claim on dietary supplements of vitamins and minerals.	"No Added Sugar" and "Without Added Sugars" are allowed if no sugar or sugar containing ingredient is added during processing. State if food is not "Low" or "Reduced Calorie". The terms "Unsweetened" and "Added Sweeteners" remain as factual statements. Claims about reducing dental caries are implied health claims. Does not include sugar alcohols.

Notes: * Except if the ingredient listed in the ingredient statement has an asterisk that refers to footnote (e.g., "* adds a trivial amount of fat").
• "Reference Amount" = serving, or amount customarily consumed.
• "Small Reference Amount" = reference amount of 30 g or less or 2 tablespoons or less (for dehydrated foods that are typically consumed when rehydrated with water or a diluent containing an insignificant amount, as defined in 21 CFR 101.9(f)(1), of all nutrients per reference amount, the per 50 g criterion refers to the prepared form of the food).
• When levels exceed: 13 g Fat, 4 g Saturated Fat, 60 mg Cholesterol, and 480 mg Sodium per reference amount, per labeled serving or, for foods with small reference amounts, per 50 g, a disclosure statement is required as part of claim (e.g., "See nutrition information for___content" with the blank filled in with nutrient(s) that exceed the prescribed levels).

SOURCE: *A Food Labeling Guide,* U.S. Food and Drug Administration, June 1999

nutrient claims as "fortified, enriched, added, extra, and plus," but in those cases, the food must be nutritionally altered.

HEALTH CLAIMS

The FDA also allows health claims on food labels. Health claims are different from "structure/function" claims found on labels of conventional food and dietary supplements. While manufacturers use health claims primarily to sell their products, the FDA believes that "these claims alert shoppers to a product's health potential by stating that certain foods or food substances—as part of an overall healthy diet—may reduce the risk of certain diseases."

Claims can be made in several ways—through third party references, such as the National Cancer Institute; via statements; by using symbols, such as a heart; and by descriptions. A health claim can use only the terms "may" or "might" in discussing the link between the nutrient and the disease; in addition, it cannot state any degree of risk reduction. Moreover, the claim must state that other factors play a role in the disease. Finally, health claims cannot be made for infants and toddlers under two years old.

Food and Drug Administration Modernization Act of 1997

In 1993 seven health claims were authorized under the 1990 NLEA. Since then, the FDA has allowed three more health claims. The Food and Drug Administration Modernization Act of 1997 (PL 105-115) provides that the process of establishing the scientific basis for health claims be expedited. It used to take more than a year to complete the process of approving a health claim because of the time required for the scientific review and the issuance of a proposed rule.

The new law allows a manufacturer to notify the FDA that it intends to use a new health claim based on an authoritative statement of one or more federal scientific bodies (for example, the National Academy of Sciences, USDA, or Institute of Medicine). The FDA has 120 days to act or make changes to the claim, after which the claim can be used.

Current Health Claims

As of June 2001, the health claims (Table 6.7) permitted by the FDA may show a link between:

• A diet with enough calcium and a lower risk of osteoporosis.

TABLE 6.7

Guide to U.S. Food and Drug Administration requirements for claiming certain health benefits on food labels

Approved claims	Food requirements	Label requirements	Model claim statements
Calcium and Osteoporosis—21 CFR 101.72	- High in calcium, - Assimilable (Bioavailable), - Supplements must disintegrate and dissolve, and - Phosphorus content cannot exceed calcium content	Indicates disease depends on many factors by listing risk factors of the disease: Gender—Female. Race—Caucasian and Asian. Age—Growing older. Primary target population: Females, Caucasian and Asian races, and teens and young adults in their bone-forming years. Additional factors necessary to reduce risk: Eating healthful meals, regular exercise. Mechanism relating calcium to osteoporosis: Optimizes peak bone mass. Foods or supplements containing more than 400 mg calcium must state that total intakes of greater than 2,000 mg calcium provide no added benefit to bone health.	Regular exercise and a healthy diet with enough calcium helps teens and young adult white and Asian women maintain good bone health and may reduce their high risk of osteoporosis later in life.
Sodium and Hypertension—21 CFR 101.74	- Low sodium	Required terms: "Sodium", "High blood pressure" Includes physician statement (Individuals with high blood pressure should consult their physicians) if claim defines high or normal blood pressure.	Diets low in sodium may reduce the risk of high blood pressure, a disease associated with many factors.
Dietary Fat and Cancer—21 CFR 101.73	- Low fat (Fish & game meats: "Extra lean")	Required terms: "Total fat" or "Fat", "Some types of cancers" or "Some cancers" Does not specify types of fats or fatty acids that may be related to risk of cancer.	Development of cancer depends on many factors. A diet low in total fat may reduce the risk of some cancers.
Dietary Saturated Fat and Cholesterol and Risk of Coronary Heart Disease—21 CFR 101.75	- Low saturated fat, - Low cholesterol, and - Low fat (Fish & game meats: "Extra lean")	Required terms: "Saturated fat and cholesterol", "Coronary heart disease" or "Heart disease" Includes physician statement (individuals with elevated blood total —or LDL—cholesterol should consult their physicians) if claim defines high or normal blood total—and LDL— cholesterol.	While many factors affect heart disease, diets low in saturated fat and cholesterol may reduce the risk of this disease.
Fiber-Containing Grain Products, Fruits, and Vegetables and Cancer—21 CFR 101.76	- A grain product, fruit, or vegetable that contains dietary fiber, - Low fat, and - Good source of dietary fiber (without fortification)	Required terms: "Fiber", "Dietary fiber", or "Total dietary fiber"; "Some types of cancer" or "Some cancers" Does not specify types of dietary fiber that may be related to risk of cancer.	Low fat diets rich in fiber-containing grain products, fruits, and vegetables may reduce the risk of some types of cancer, a disease associated with many factors.
Fruits, Vegetables and Grain Products that contain Fiber, particularly Soluble Fiber, and Risk of Coronary Heart Disease—21 CFR 101.77	- A fruit, vegetable, or grain product that contains fiber, - Low saturated fat, - Low cholesterol, - Low fat, - At least 0.6 grams of soluble fiber per RA (without fortification), and - Soluble fiber content provided on label	Required terms: "Fiber", "Dietary fiber", "Some types of dietary fiber", "Some dietary fibers", or "Some fibers"; "Saturated fat" and "Cholesterol"; "Heart disease" or "Coronary heart disease" Includes physician statement ("Individuals with elevated blood total—or LDL—cholesterol should consult their physicians") if claim defines high or normal blood total —and LDL—cholesterol.	Diets low in saturated fat and cholesterol and rich in fruits, vegetables, and grain products that contain some types of dietary fiber, particularly soluble fiber, may reduce the risk of heart disease, a disease associated with many factors.

- A diet low in sodium and a reduced risk of high blood pressure.

- A diet low in total fat and a reduced risk of some cancers.

- A diet low in saturated fat and cholesterol and a reduced risk of coronary heart disease.

- A diet rich in fiber-containing grain products, fruits, and vegetables and a reduced risk of some cancers.

- A diet rich in fruits, vegetables, and grain products that contain fiber and a reduced risk of coronary heart disease.

TABLE 6.7

Guide to U.S. Food and Drug Administration requirements for claiming certain health benefits on food labels [CONTINUED]

Approved claims	Food requirements	Label requirements	Model claim statements
Fruits and Vegetables and Cancer—21 CFR 101.78	- A fruit or vegetable, - Low fat, and - Good source (without fortification) of at least one of the following: Vitamin A, Vitamin C, or Dietary fiber	Required terms: "Fiber", "Dietary fiber", or "Total dietary fiber"; "Total fat" or "Fat"; "Some types of cancer" or "Some cancers" Characterizes fruits and vegetables as "Foods that are low in fat and may contain Vitamin A, Vitamin C, and dietary fiber." Characterizes specific food as a "Good source" of one or more of the following: Dietary fiber, Vitamin A, or Vitamin C. Does not specify types of fats or fatty acids or types of dietary fiber that may be related to risk of cancer.	Low fat diets rich in fruits and vegetables (foods that are low in fat and may contain dietary fiber, Vitamin A, or Vitamin C) may reduce the risk of some types of cancer, a disease associated with many factors. Broccoli is high in vitamin A and C, and it is a good source of dietary fiber.
Folate and Neural Tube Defects—21 CFR 101.79	-"Good source" of folate (at least 40 mg folate per serving) - Dietary supplements, or foods in conventional food form that are naturally good sources of folate (i.e., only non-fortified food in conventional food form) - The claim shall not be made on products that contain more than 100% of the RDI for vitamin A as retinol or preformed vitamin A or vitamin D. - Dietary supplements shall meet USP standards for disintegration and dissolution or otherwise bioavailable. -Amount of folate required in N.L.	Required terms: Terms that specify the relationship (e.g., women who are capable of becoming pregnant and who consume adequate amounts of folate) "Folate", "folic acid", "folacin","folate, a B vitamin", "folic acid, a B vitamin," "folacin, a B vitamin," "neural tube defects", "birth defects, spinal bifida, or anencephaly", "birth defects of the brain or spinal cord—anencephaly or spinal bifida", "spinal bifida or anencephaly, birth defects of the brain or spinal cord". Must also include information on the multifactorial nature of neural tube defects, and the safe upper limit of daily intake.	Healthful diets with adequate folate may reduce a woman's risk of having a child with a brain or spinal cord defect.
Dietary Sugar Alcohol and Dental Caries—21 CFR 101.80	- Sugar free. - The sugar alcohol must be xylitol, sorbitol, mannitol, maltitol, isomalt, lactitol, hydrogenated starch hydrolysates, hydrogenated glucose syrups, erythritol, or a combination. - When a fermentable carbohydrate is present, the food must not lower plaque pH below 5.7.	Required terms: "does not promote," "may reduce the risk of", "useful [or is useful] in not promoting" or "expressly [or is expressly] for not promoting" dental caries; "sugar alcohol" or "sugar alcohols" or the name or names of the sugar alcohols, e.g., sorbitol; "dental caries" or "tooth decay." Includes statement that frequent between meal consumption of foods high in sugars and starches can promote tooth decay. Packages with less than 15 square inches of surface area available for labeling may use a shortened claim.	**Full claim:** Frequent between-meal consumption of foods high in sugars and starches promotes tooth decay. The sugar alcohols in [name of food] do not promote tooth decay. **Shortened claim (on small packages only):** Does not promote tooth decay.
Soluble Fiber from Certain Foods and Risk of Coronary Heart Disease—21 CFR 101.81	- Low saturated fat, - Low cholesterol, - Low fat, - Include either (1) one or more eligible sources of whole oats, containing at least 0.75 g whole oat soluble fiber per RA; or (2) psyllium seed husk containing at least 1.7 g of psyllium husk soluble fiber per RA, and - Amount of soluble fiber per RA declared in nutrition label. **Eligible Source of Soluble Fiber:** Beta glucan soluble fiber from oat bran, rolled oats (or oatmeal), and whole oat flour. Oat bran must provide at least 5.5% glucan soluble fiber, rolled oats must provide at least 4% glucan soluble fiber, and whole oat flour must provide at least 4% glucan soluble fiber or psyllium husk with purity of no less than 95%.	Required terms: "Heart disease" or "coronary heart disease"; "Soluble fiber" qualified by either "psyllium seed husk" or the name of the eligible source of whole oat soluble fiber; "saturated fat" and "cholesterol." Daily dietary intake of the soluble fiber source necessary to reduce the risk of CHD and the contribution one serving of the product makes to this level of intake. **Additional Required Label Statement:** Foods bearing a psyllium seed husk health claim must also bear a label statement concerning the need to consume them with adequate amounts of fluids; e.g., "NOTICE: This food should be eaten with at least a full glass of liquid. Eating this product without enough liquid may cause choking. Do not eat this product if you have difficulty in swallowing." (21 CFR 101.17(f))	Soluble fiber from foods such as [name of soluble fiber source, and, if desired, name of food product], as part of a diet low in saturated fat and cholesterol, may reduce the risk of heart disease. A serving of [name of food product] supplies __ grams of the [necessary daily dietary intake for the benefit] soluble fiber from [name of soluble fiber source] necessary per day to have this effect.

TABLE 6.7

Guide to U.S. Food and Drug Administration requirements for claiming certain health benefits on food labels [CONTINUED]

Approved claims	Food requirements	Label requirements	Model claim statements
Soy Protein and Risk of Coronary Heart Disease—21 CFR 101.82	- At least 6.25 g soy protein per RA, - Low saturated fat, - Low cholesterol, and - Low fat (except that foods made from whole soybeans that contain no fat in addition to that inherent in the whole soybean are exempt from the "low fat" requirement)	Required terms: "Heart disease" or "coronary heart disease"; "Soy protein"; "Saturated fat" and "cholesterol" Claim specifies daily dietary intake levels of soy protein associated with reduced risk. Claim specifies amount of soy protein in a serving of food.	(1) 25 grams of soy protein a day, as part of a diet low in saturated fat and cholesterol, may reduce the risk of heart disease. A serving of [name of food] supplies __ grams of soy protein. (2) Diets low in saturated fat and cholesterol that include 25 grams of soy protein a day may reduce the risk of heart disease. One serving of [name of food] provides __ grams of soy protein.
Plant Sterol/Stanol Esters and Risk of Coronary Heart Disease—21 CFR 101.83	- At least 0.65 g plant sterol esters per RA of spreads and salad dressing, or - At least 1.7 g plant stanol esters per RA of spreads, salad dressings, snack bars, and dietary supplements. - Low saturated fat, - Low cholesterol, and - Spreads and salad dressings that exceed 13 g fat per 50 g must bear the statement "see nutrition information for fat content" Salad dressings are exempted from the minimum 10% DV nutrient requirement (see General Criteria below)	Required terms: "May" or "might" reduce the risk of CHD; "Heart disease" or "coronary heart disease"; "Plant sterol esters" or "plant stanol esters"; except "vegetable oil" may replace the term "plant" if vegetable oil is the sole source of the sterol/stanol ester. Claim specifies plant sterol/stanol esters are part of a diet low in saturated fat and cholesterol. Claim does not attribute any degree of CHD risk reduction. Claim specifies the daily dietary intake of plant sterol or stanol esters necessary to reduce CHD risk, and the amount provided per serving. Claim specifies that plant sterol or stanol esters should be consumed with two different meals each a day.	(1) Foods containing at least 0.65 gram per serving of vegetable oil sterol esters, eaten twice a day with meals for a daily total intake of at least 1.3 grams, as part of a diet low in saturated fat and cholesterol, may reduce the risk of heart disease. A serving of [name of food] supplies __ grams of vegetable oil sterol esters. (2) Diets low in saturated fat and cholesterol that include two servings of foods that provide a daily total of at least 3.4 grams of plant stanol esters in two meals may reduce the risk of heart disease. A serving of [name of food] supplies __ grams of plant stanol esters.

CLAIMS AUTHORIZED BASED ON AUTHORITATIVE STATEMENTS BY FEDERAL SCIENTIFIC BODIES

Approved claims	Food requirements	Label requirements	Model claim statements
Whole Grain Foods and Risk of Heart Disease and Certain Cancers—Docket No. 99P-2209	- Contains 51 percent or more whole grain ingredients by weight per RA, and - Dietary fiber content at least: • 3.0 g per RA of 55 g • 2.8 g per RA of 50 g • 2.5 g per RA of 45 g • 1.7 g per RA of 35 g - Low fat	Required wording of the claim: "Diets rich in whole grain foods and other plant foods and low in total fat, saturated fat, and cholesterol may reduce the risk of heart disease and some cancers."	NA
Potassium and the Risk of High Blood Pressure and Stroke—Docket No. 00Q-1582	- Good source of potassium, - Low sodium, - Low total fat, - Low saturated fat, and - Low cholesterol	Required wording of the claim: "Diets containing foods that are a good source of potassium and that are low in sodium may reduce the risk of high blood pressure and stroke."	NA

GENERAL CRITERIA ALL CLAIMS MUST MEET

All information must appear in one place without intervening material (reference statement permitted). Only information on the value that intake or reduced intake, as part of a total dietary pattern, may have on a disease or health-related condition is permitted. Enables public to understand information provided and significance of information in the context of a total daily diet. Must be complete, truthful, and not misleading. Food contains, without fortification, 10% or more of the Daily Value for one of six nutrients (dietary supplements excepted):

Vitamin A 500 IU	Calcium 100 mg
Vitamin C 6 mg	Protein 5 g
Iron 1.8 mg	Fiber 2.5 g

Not represented for infants or toddlers less than 2 years of age. Uses "may" or "might" to express relationship between substance and disease. Does not quantify any degree of risk reduction. Indicates disease depends on many factors.

Food contains less than the specified levels of four disqualifying nutrients:

Disqualifying Nutrients	Foods	Main Dishes	Meal Products
Fat	13 g	19.5 g	26 g
Saturated Fat	4 g	6 g	8 g
Cholesterol	60 mg	90 mg	120 mg
Sodium	480 mg	720 mg	960 mg

Abbreviations: RA = reference amount, IU = International Units

SOURCE: *A Food Labeling Guide*, U.S. Food and Drug Administration, June 1999

- A diet rich in fruits and vegetables and a reduced risk of some cancers.

- Folic acid and a decreased risk of neural tube defect during pregnancy.

- Dietary sugar alcohols and a reduced risk of dental caries.

- Soluble fiber from certain foods, such as whole oats and psyllium seed husk, as part of a diet low in saturated fat and cholesterol, and a reduced risk of heart disease.

- Soy protein and the risk of coronary heart disease.

- Plant sterol/stanol esters and the risk of coronary heart disease.

- Whole grain foods and the risk of heart disease and certain cancers.

- Potassium and the risk of high blood pressure and stroke.

In addition, the FDA identified fat, saturated fat, cholesterol, and sodium as risk nutrients and set specific levels per serving of these "disqualifying nutrients." Single-item foods bearing a health claim must contain 20 percent or less of the Daily Value of fat (13 g), saturated fat (4 g), cholesterol (60 mg), and sodium (480 mg). For example, whole milk, which is rich in calcium, is not permitted to bear a calcium-osteoporosis claim on its nutrition label because its fat content exceeds the disqualifying levels. (See Table 6.7 footnotes for other FDA-specified levels of disqualifying nutrients for main dishes and meal products.)

OTHER LABEL CLAIMS

According to the NLEA, in order to use the claim "percent fat free," a product must also be a low-fat or a fat-free food. The claim must also accurately reflect the amount of fat present in 100 grams of the food. In other words, if a food contains 2.5 grams of fat per 50 grams, the product claim must be "95 percent fat free."

A "healthy" food must be low in total fat and saturated fat and contain limited amounts of sodium and cholesterol. If it is a single-serving food, it must provide at least 10 percent of one or more of vitamins A or C, iron, calcium, protein, or fiber. "Healthy" meal-type products, such as frozen dinners, must provide 10 percent of two or three of these nutrients. These nutrients would have to occur naturally in the food; they cannot be added. Moreover, the sodium content cannot exceed 360 mg per serving for single-serving foods and 480 mg for meal-type foods.

The NLEA allows manufacturers to reduce the fat content of certain foods and call them "low fat" or "light" as long as those foods are still nutritionally equivalent to the original product. For example, sour cream can be called "light" if the fat content is reduced to 9 percent (from the regular 18 percent) and has vitamin A added to replace the amount lost when the fat was removed. If the manufacturer does not replace the vitamin A, the product must be labeled "imitation light sour cream."

"IMPLIED" CLAIMS ARE PROHIBITED

An "implied" claim occurs when a product label appears to confer a certain health benefit through a nutrition claim. The FDA prohibits this. For example, if a product advertises that it is "made with canola oil," it is implying that the product is low in saturated fat. To carry that claim, however, the food itself, not just the canola oil that went into the recipe, must actually be low in saturated fat.

Exceptions

Certain statements that do not fall under the "implied" claim prohibition and therefore are allowed, include:

- Avoidance claims for religious or food-intolerance reasons, such as the term "milk/dairy-free."

- Statements about non-nutritive ingredients, such as "no preservatives" or "no artificial colors."

- Added-value statements, such as "contains real fruit" or "made with real butter."

- Statements of identity, such as "corn oil margarine" or "Colombian coffee."

LABELING FOR FAT-REDUCED MILK

Milk occupies a significant place in the American diet, providing a large portion of saturated fat (after cheese and beef). Replacing full-fat milk with lower-fat or skim milk would significantly lower an individual's saturated-fat intake. Eight ounces of full-fat milk provides 26 percent of the Daily Value for saturated fat, compared to skim milk, which provides none.

In January 1998 the FDA ruled that the labeling of fat-reduced milk and milk products must follow the same specifications for other foods reduced in fat. In making milk labeling consistent with that of other food products, the FDA aimed to give consumers more accurate, consistent information. For example, low-fat milk, or 1 percent milk, is required to have the same fat content as any low-fat dessert. The FDA allows these low-fat food items to provide no more than three grams of fat per serving.

Milk products with lower-fat contents are required to be nutritionally equivalent to full-fat (whole) milk and provide at least the same amount of fat-soluble vitamins A and D as full-fat milk. These two vitamins are lost when milk fat is removed or reduced and are replaced later in the process.

Dietary Impact

Nutrition experts believe that the new milk labeling will not only help consumers differentiate between reduced-fat milk and low-fat milk, it might also encourage them to switch from the former to the latter. Two-percent milk has almost twice the amount of total fat as 1-percent milk.

NUTRITION INFORMATION ON FRESH FOODS

In 1991, in accordance with the NLEA, the FDA established guidelines for voluntary nutrition labeling on fresh fruits, vegetables, and fish. The program will remain voluntary only if at least 60 percent of retailers continue to participate in the program. According to the FDA, a 1996 survey showed that more than 70 percent of U.S. food retailers participated in the voluntary point-of-purchase nutrition information program.

Currently, nutrition labeling is available for the 20 most frequently eaten raw fruits, vegetables, and fish. Grocers can convey nutrition information through stickers, posters, brochures, leaflets, or any other method as long as the information is readily available to consumers. Although participation is voluntary, the FDA regulates the information offered. The information must include serving size; calories per serving; amount of protein; total carbohydrate, total fat, and sodium; and percent of the Reference Daily Intakes for iron, calcium, and vitamins A and C per serving.

The Food Safety and Inspection Service (FSIS) of the USDA has established a similar voluntary program for raw meat and poultry. The program includes major cuts of raw single-ingredient meat and poultry products. As with raw fruits, vegetables, and fish, nutrition information may be displayed on posters, brochures, and other point-of-purchase materials, as long as they are located near the food. The information may also be included on the package label. The information must include serving size based on raw or cooked weight; calories per serving; calories from total fat per serving; amount per serving (by weight and by Percent Daily Values) for total fat, saturated fat, cholesterol, sodium, total carbohydrate, and dietary fiber; amount by weight of sugars and protein; and Percent Daily Values per serving for vitamins A and C, calcium, and iron.

NUTRITION LABELING EXEMPTIONS

Under the NLEA some foods are exempt from nutrition labeling. These include:

- food served for immediate consumption such as that served in hospital cafeterias and airplanes, and that sold by food-service vendors—for example, mall cookie counters, sidewalk vendors, and vending machines.

- ready-to-eat food that is not for immediate consumption but is prepared primarily on-site—for example, bakery, deli, and candy store items.

- food shipped in bulk, as long as it is not for sale in that form to consumers.

- medical foods, such as those used to address the nutritional needs of patients with certain diseases.

- plain coffee and tea, some spices, and other foods that contain no significant amounts of any nutrients.

SHOPPERS READ FOOD LABELS

The Food Marketing Institute, in *Trends in the United States—Consumer Attitudes and the Supermarket 2000* (Washington, D.C., 2000), asked shoppers how often they read food labels for nutrition and ingredient information. Nearly three-quarters (70 percent) looked for and purchased products labeled as "low fat," and over half looked for and purchased products labels as "low cholesterol," "natural," and "low salt." Consumers with more education, higher incomes, and those over 40 years old were the most likely to read nutrition labels.

Among the factors in deciding to purchase a food item for the first time, health claims were third most important after price and brand name.

CHAPTER 7
FOOD SAFETY

FOODBORNE ILLNESSES

In the United States, where food is often sold prepackaged and has government seals of inspection, consumers expect food to be safe. However, outbreaks of foodborne illness do occur, and have caused public concern about the safety of food. Today, the public realizes that any kind of food can be tainted with bacteria at any point, from the processing plant to the consumer's kitchen.

In 1993 three children and one adult died and many more got sick from contaminated hamburgers in the Pacific Northwest. In 1998 a juice maker agreed to what is believed to be the biggest settlement involving food poisoning from ingestion of fresh food. The families of five children who suffered severely from drinking fresh-squeezed apple juice may have received as much as $15 million. A total of 70 people got ill from this food-poisoning outbreak, including an infant who died.

The USDA estimates that 76 million illnesses, including 5,200 deaths, occur from food poisoning each year, resulting in an annual cost of $6.9 billion. In 1998, President Bill Clinton signed an executive order establishing a President's Council on Food Safety.

FOODBORNE PATHOGENS

At least 30 pathogens (harmful bacteria, viruses, chemicals, and parasites) are associated with foodborne illness. Bacterial pathogens are the most commonly identified cause of foodborne illnesses. Chemical pathogens are usually natural toxins in food and in such metals as copper and cadmium. Viruses, such as hepatitis A, are transmitted by infected food handlers or through contact with sewage. Parasites can also grow in host animals. For example, *Trichinella* is found in raw or undercooked pork.

Bacterial Pathogens

According to the Centers for Disease Control and Prevention (CDC), the federal agency primarily responsible for monitoring the incidence of foodborne illnesses, ailments resulting from bacterial pathogens can cause serious complications beyond the immediate food-poisoning crisis. Arthritis, organ failures, stillbirths, and other complications may follow an episode of food poisoning. (See Table 7.1.)

CAMPYLOBACTER JEJUNI. The CDC reports that *Campylobacter jejuni* is the most common bacterial cause of diarrhea in the developed world. The bacterium can infect all age groups, but it affects children under one year old the most.

Every year 2 to 10 million Americans suffer from *Campylobacter* infection. It is caused mainly by raw poultry and beef, unpasteurized milk, polluted water, and pets. The illness lasts 2 to 10 days, causing diarrhea, fever, headache, and chills. Between 200 and 730 victims die from campylobacteriosis annually. (See Table 7.2.)

CAMPYLOBACTER-ASSOCIATED GUILLAIN-BARRÉ SYNDROME (GBS). In the United States, Guillain-Barré Syndrome, characterized by nerve damage that may develop into paralysis, is currently the leading cause of paralysis from a disease.

Medical studies worldwide have found that 20 to 40 percent of Guillain-Barré Syndrome (GBS) patients had been afflicted with *Campylobacter* infection one to three weeks before exhibiting GBS symptoms. *Campylobacter*, the leading bacterial cause of foodborne illnesses in the United States, has significantly increased the instances, and, therefore, the financial costs of these ailments. Almost all afflicted individuals need hospitalization, and some suffer relapses. About 20 percent of GBS patients become significantly disabled, and 2 percent die.

ESCHERICHIA COLI (E. COLI) O157:H7. *E. coli* O157:H7 food poisoning occurs when meat has come in contact with animal feces carrying the bacterium, usually

TABLE 7.1

Some foodborne pathogens that can cause serious illnesses

Foodborne pathogen	Serious illnesses that can result	Foods in which pathogens have been found
Bacteria		
Campylobacter	Arthritis, blood poisoning, Guillain-Barre syndrome (paralysis), chronic diarrhea, meningitis, and inflammation of the heart, gallbladder, colon, and pancreas	Poultry, raw milk, and meat
E. coli O157:H7	HUS,[a] which is associated with kidney failure and neurologic disorders; and other illnesses	Meat, especially ground beef; raw milk; and produce
Listeria	Meningitis, blood poisoning, stillbirths, and other disorders	Soft cheese, other dairy products, meat, poultry, seafood, fruits, and vegetables
Salmonella	Reactive arthritis, blood poisoning, Reiter's disease (inflammation of joints, eye membranes, and urinary tract) and inflammation of the pancreas, spleen, colon, gallbladder, thyroid, and heart	Poultry, meat, eggs, dairy products, seafood, fruits, and vegetables
Shigella	Reiter's disease, HUS, pneumonia, blood poisoning, neurologic disorders, and inflammation of the spleen	Salads, milk and dairy products, and produce
Vibrio vulnificus	Blood poisoning	Seafood
Yersinia enterocolitica	Reiter's disease, pnemonia, and inflammation of vertebrae, lymphatic glands, liver, and spleen	Pork and dairy products
Parasites		
Toxoplasma gondii	Central nervous system disorders	Meat, primarily pork
Trichinella spiralis	Heart and neurologic disorders	Pork

[a]Hemolytic-uremic syndrome.

SOURCE: "Some Foodborne Pathogens That Can Cause Serious Illnesses" in *Food Safety: Information on Foodborne Illnesses,* U.S. General Accounting Office, Washington, D.C., 1996

at the slaughterhouse or at the packing plant. People have billions of the bacteria in their intestines, and many strains of *E. coli* are harmless. However, the CDC estimates that between 20,000 and 40,000 Americans are infected with *E. coli* O157:H7 disease each year. About 50 to 100 die. (See Table 7.2.)

E. coli O157:H7 infection tends to strike the very young or very old and those with weak or immature immune systems. Most cases are mild to moderate, occurring two to five days after eating contaminated food. Diarrhea can last six to eight days, and bloody diarrhea occurs in about half of these cases.

Less than 5 percent (1,000 to 2,000) of *E. coli* O157:H7 cases develop into hemolytic uremic syndrome, a disease characterized by red blood-cell destruction, kidney failure, seizures, and strokes. Most cases occur among children under five years old, although the frail elderly may also be at risk. Death results in about 29 to 58 cases annually. (See Table 7.2.) The CDC reports that, as of 2000, *E. coli* O157:H7 infection was the leading cause of acute kidney failure in children.

While raw or undercooked ground beef is the most likely source of *E. coli* O157:H7 contamination, the bacterium has also been traced to unpasteurized apple cider, unpasteurized milk, water, some fresh produce, turkey roll, and mayonnaise. The infection can spread from person to person.

In 1997 the U.S. Department of Agriculture (USDA) recalled 25 million pounds of beef believed contaminated with *E. coli* O157:H7. This was the largest meat recall in U.S. history, and, as a result, the Nebraska plant where the beef had been processed was shut down.

LISTERIA MONOCYTOGENES. About 1,092 to 1,860 cases of listeriosis occur each year, with 270 to 510 victims dying (Table 7.2.) Soft and semi-soft cheese, processed meats, undercooked chicken, and delicatessen salads are the usual sources of contamination. Unlike other bacteria, *Listeria* thrives in cold temperatures and can grow under refrigeration.

Listeriosis may be mild or severe. The symptoms of milder cases are sudden fever, headache, and other characteristics resembling influenza. The infection may last three to four weeks. A pregnant woman afflicted with Listeria may pass the infection to her fetus, resulting in stillbirth or mental retardation in the baby. Listeria can travel from the gastrointestinal tract to the brain, causing meningitis. Blood poisoning may also occur. (See Table 7.1.)

SALMONELLA. Only a handful of the more than 2,000 types of *Salmonella* cause food poisoning, but an estimated 800,000 to 4 million *Salmonella* illnesses occur every year in the United States. About 1,000 to 2,000 of those infected die. (See Table 7.2.) The illness begins within 6 to 72 hours of infection. The symptoms include severe diarrhea, nausea, vomiting, and fever, lasting from one to two days.

Raw or undercooked chicken, beef, and eggs are the foods most likely to be contaminated with *Salmonella*, but it has also been found in unpasteurized milk, cheese, chocolate, fruits, and vegetables. People who have come in contact with infected stools can spread the infection. Most people know to take precautions with raw chicken, but recently the organism has flourished because it can now be transmitted from hens to the yolks of intact eggs.

"MAD COW DISEASE". In 1996 Europeans were frightened by a small outbreak of brain disease in Great Britain that resembled Creutzfeldt-Jakob disease (CJD). CJD, a very rare degenerative condition, usually affects people over 65, causing dementia and muscular contractions. The new variant CJD, a fatal illness, has been linked to bovine spongiform encephalopathy, more commonly known as "mad cow disease."

"Mad cow disease" first plagued cows in Great Britain in 1986, causing animals to develop spongy areas in their brains, stagger, behave strangely, and die by the thousands. It was believed that the disease was caused by infected, ground-up animal parts used as animal feed. Consumers were warned to stay away from beef, and 1.7 million cattle were destroyed in an effort to eliminate the disease. "Mad cow disease" has been confirmed among native-born cattle in Belgium, France, Switzerland, Germany, and Spain. So far it has not occurred in the United States, though some livestock has been slaughtered under suspicion of the disease.

In 1999 the London School of Hygiene and Tropical Medicine, which tracks the new variant CJD, reported that in the last quarter of 1998, nine people in Great Britain had died from the disease, up from no more than four cases per three-month period in the past three years. The human version of "mad cow disease" was first recognized in 1995. By the end of 1998, 39 Britons had died from the disease. Early in 1999 nearly 174,000 cows came down with "mad cow disease" in Great Britain. More than four million cattle were destroyed to arrest the infection, and slaughters continued during 2000 and 2001.

COMPUTER TRACKING OF FOODBORNE ILLNESSES

In May 1998 the federal government introduced a new computer tracking system to expedite the identification of foodborne illnesses throughout the United States. The PulseNet computer network links the CDC, the Food

and Drug Administration (FDA), the USDA, four laboratories, and state health departments.

When an outbreak of a foodborne illness occurs, the agencies identify the pathogen quickly, using the DNA of the bacteria in the tainted food and in afflicted individuals. The DNA code of the bacteria is then transmitted throughout the 50 states to determine if a similar illness has occurred in another site. Protective safeguards, such as a product recall, can then be initiated immediately.

COSTS OF FOODBORNE ILLNESSES

Economists use two methods to estimate the financial costs of foodborne illnesses. The labor market approach

TABLE 7.2

Seven pathogens found in food and nonfood sources

Pathogen, acute illness, and complication	Estimated total annual		Estimated share foodborne
	Cases	Deaths	
	Number		*Percent*
Bacteria:			
Campylobacter jejuni or *coli*–			
Campylobacteriosis	2,000,000–10,000,000	200–730	55–70
Guillain–Barré Syndrome	532–3,830	10–76	55–70
Subtotal	N/A	210–806	N/A
Clostridium perfringens–			
C. perfringens intoxications	10,000	100	100
Escherichia coli O157:H7–			
E. coli O157:H7 disease	20,000–40,000	50–100	80
Hemolytic uremic syndrome[1]	1,000–2,000	29–58	80
Subtotal	N/A	79–158	N/A
Listeria monocytogenes[2]–			
Listeriosis	1,092–1,860	270–510	85–95
Complications	26–43	0	85–95
Subtotal	N/A	270–510	N/A
Salmonella (non-typhoid)–			
Salmonellosis	800,000–4,000,000	1,000–2,000	87–96
Staphylococcus aureus–			
S. aureus intoxications	8,900,000	2,670	17
Parasite:			
Toxoplasma gondii[3]–			
Toxoplasmosis	520	80	50
Complications	3,120	0	50
Subtotal	N/A[4]	80	N/A
Total	**11,700,000–23,000,000**	**4,400–6,300**	**N/A**

Notes: N/A = Not applicable. Subtotal and totals may not add due to rounding. Totals are rounded down to reflect the uncertainty of the estimates. Nonfood sources include drinking or swimming in contaminated water and contact with infected people or animals.
[1] Kidney failure.
[2] Includes only hospitalized patients because of data limitations.
[3] Includes only toxoplasmosis cases related to fetuses and newborn children who may become blind or mentally retarded. Does not include all other cases of toxoplasmosis. Another high-risk group for this parasite is the immunocompromised, such as patients with AIDS.
[4] Of the 4,000 infections from this parasite each year, 520 develop acute illness and later die prematurely or develop some degree of chronic complication because of the illness, and 2,680 do not have noticeable acute illness at birth but develop complications by age 17. Therefore, a total of 3,200 develop either acute illness, chronic complication, or both.

SOURCE: Jean C. Buzby and Tanya Roberts, "Guillain-Barré Syndrome Increases Foodborne Disease Costs," in *Food Review,* Vol. 20, Issue 3, September-December 1997

estimates the statistical value of a life by using records that show consumers' willingness to pay to reduce the risks of death and poor health. This is based on labor market data indicating how much increased salary employers must offer workers to take a job with some injury risk. This method values the cost of a premature death at $5 million.

The human capital approach estimates the value of lost productivity (loss of income from death or disability). Lost productivity is calculated using a combination of lost income estimates and willingness-to-pay estimates. On this basis, the statistical value of a life tends to range from $15,000 to $1.9 million, depending on age. Jean C. Buzby and Tanya Roberts, in "Guillain-Barré Syndrome Increases Foodborne Disease Costs" (*FoodReview,* Washington, D.C., Vol. 20, Issue 3, September-December 1997), based the estimated costs of foodborne illnesses on the human capital approach. In 1996 dollars, the cost of a premature death, depending on age, was between $15,000 and $2,037,000.

The authors noted that both methods undervalued the true costs of foodborne illnesses to society because they mainly included medical costs and lost productivity. Total costs would be higher if the expenses resulting from complications, such as arthritis or meningitis, were added. The costs would also increase if societal costs, such as pain and suffering, travel to medical care, and lost leisure time, were included.

In 1999 the CDC reported an estimated 13.8 million cases of foodborne illnesses and approximately 18,000 deaths linked to these illnesses. The difference in this estimate and the one made by the USDA is attributable to the difficulty in determining the annual total cases of foodborne illnesses and associated deaths. People who experience food poisoning often do not see a doctor. If they do, they might not have a stool culture taken; and if a culture is submitted for testing, the lab test might not find the pathogen. Furthermore, even if the pathogen is identified, it may not be reported to the CDC.

FOOD SAFETY PRECAUTIONS

There are a number of precautions consumers should take to minimize the chances of foodborne illness. The following includes general rules for food handling, storage, and consumption:

- When shopping, do not buy anything you will not use before the use-by or sell-by date.

- Refrigerate or freeze perishables, ready-to-eat foods, and leftovers as soon as possible. Freeze fresh meat and fish immediately if you will not use them within a few days.

- Thaw frozen foods in the refrigerator or microwave, not on the kitchen counter. When marinating food, keep it in the refrigerator.

- Wash your hands with hot soapy water before and after food preparation. Also, wash your hands after using the bathroom, changing diapers, and handling pets.

- When preparing raw meats, keep knives and cutting boards separate from other ingredients and wash them thoroughly with hot water and soap. If possible, use separate cutting boards for fresh produce and for raw meats and fish. Never brush a marinade that has been in contact with raw meet on cooked meat. Wash counter tops with hot soapy water.

- Buy only clean, uncracked eggs, keep them refrigerated, and avoid eating raw or undercooked eggs. Make mayonnaise and Caesar salad dressings with egg substitutes or pasteurized eggs. Do not eat raw cake batter or cookie dough.

- Wash all fruits and vegetables before eating, including those that will be peeled.

- Do not eat hamburgers that are pink in the center or steaks that are not thoroughly cooked.

REGULATING FOOD SAFETY

Food safety is a growing problem, especially because the pool of people at risk grows as the population ages and the numbers of people with illnesses or conditions that suppress the immune systems (AIDS, organ transplant patients, etc.) increase. An aging population also means greater concern about the chronic effects of both microbial and chemical contaminants (pesticides). These may have long-term effects that only become apparent with longer life spans.

Several federal agencies are responsible for food safety in the United States. The USDA inspects meat, poultry, and egg products. The FDA has regulatory responsibility for the rest of the food products, while the Environmental Protection Agency (EPA) establishes the levels of pesticide residues that can be tolerated by humans.

In 1994 the USDA established a requirement for labels with handling instructions on raw or partially cooked meat and poultry. The labels were designed to reduce the risk of foodborne illness attributable to unsafe handling, preparation, and storage.

Also in 1994 FDA Commissioner David Kessler turned to the National Aeronautics and Space Administration (NASA) to copy its program for ensuring safe food. NASA knew it would be disastrous to have an astronaut in outer space with food poisoning, so it developed the Hazard Analysis and Critical Control Points (HACCP) program to prevent food poisoning before it could occur. Instead of looking for bacteria in finished products, manufacturing plants would have to identify the points where infection is most likely to occur ("Critical Control

Points"—CCP) and design a plan to prevent contamination, keeping careful records to document their efforts.

For example, poultry producers would have to certify that feces are not rubbed into the bird's skin as it is defeathered, that the chill tank is not a "fecal soup," and that the birds are chilled quickly enough to prevent the growth of bacteria. The HACCP program has been adapted and applied to meat and fish processing.

Meat Regulations

Before the present system, the USDA used organoleptic inspection to test for food safety—inspectors judged the safety of the meat through what they could see, feel, and smell. While organoleptic inspection could identify grossly visible lesions or diseases, it could not identify microbial pathogens, the cause of today's principal health risks. In poultry inspections, for example, the inspector had approximately two seconds to visually examine the inside and outside surfaces of each bird and feel the eviscerated (removed) internal organs.

In July 1996 the government instituted new regulations for meat inspections. Some of the new rules took effect immediately, while others would go into effect after several years. The main elements of the regulations included the following:

- No processing plant would be allowed to exceed the average level of salmonella contamination that existed before the regulations. For chicken, the acceptable bacteria level was 20 percent; for turkey, it was 49 percent.

- Processors would be required to test all their products for *E. coli* O157:H7, which is a reliable indicator of fecal contamination. Processors would not be required to eliminate the bacteria altogether but would have to keep contamination below specific levels.

- Every processing plant would be required to identify critical points along the chain where products could become contaminated. The plants would check for contamination at each point from the time when the product is received from the farm to when it leaves for the grocery store.

- All plants would have to adopt written plans to prevent contamination. These would include items such as the method the plant uses to ensure that surface bacteria from the animal's skin does not contaminate the meat.

The USDA estimated the regulations would cost the meat industry about $80 million a year and would cost consumers one-tenth of a cent per pound of meat. The USDA further estimated that every 1 percent reduction in illness caused by unsafe handling and cooking of raw meat would result in annual societal savings of between $38.8 million and $43.3 million. The benefits would come from savings in medical costs, time lost from work, and loss of life.

Seafood Regulations

The FDA also developed an HACCP (Hazard Analysis and Critical Control Points) program for the seafood industry, which took effect in early 1996. Seafood contaminants include the deadly *Vibrio vulnificus*, which kills half of those it infects, as well as other bacteria, viruses, natural toxins, parasites, and chemicals. The HACCP program consists of seven steps for seafood:

- Identify the likely health hazards to consumers in a given product.

- Identify the Critical Control Points where there is a risk of contamination.

- Establish safety measures to prevent a hazard from occurring.

- Monitor the system to ensure that the safety measures are working.

- Establish the appropriate remedy if monitoring shows a problem.

- Establish detailed record keeping to document the steps taken and the remedies put in place.

- Verify that the control system is working.

The FDA estimated that implementing this program would cost an average of $24,000 for small firms (annual sales of less than $1 million) and $23,400 for large plants. The costs are greater for small plants because most of them do not already have HACCP-type controls in place. In subsequent years, the plan would cost small plants about $14,700 a year and large plants, about $15,700. The costs will be passed on to consumers in the form of higher prices. The FDA estimates that between 6,500 and 19,000 cases of seafood-caused illnesses or, in some cases, deaths could be averted under the HACCP program at a value of between $15 million and $75 million a year.

Food Additive Regulations

Whole foods, as opposed to functional foods (foods that contain a substance or substances that, manufacturers claim, perform a function in the body), are generally not required to undergo pre-market review or approval by the FDA, but they are subject to postmarket surveillance for adulteration. The FDA, however, can regulate any "added" substance (additive) that does not naturally occur in a food if it "may" cause harm. The FDA can remove a food item if there is a reasonable possibility that a harmful substance has been added to it. Food manufacturers are responsible for proving that additives are safe before their products go to market. Manufacturers of food and color additives must demonstrate a reasonable certainty that consumers will not be harmed as a result of the intended use of an additive. Furthermore, if any food additive is found to induce cancer in animals or people, its use will not be approved.

EXEMPTIONS. Two categories of substances are exempt from food additive regulations. Prior-sanctioned substances are substances that were approved by the FDA or the USDA before 1958. "Generally recognized as safe" (GRAS) substances are substances that "experts qualified by scientific training and experience" have generally recognized as safe when used as intended in food. For example, salt, pepper, vinegar, vegetable oil, spices, and natural flavors, as well as some preservatives and sweeteners, are legally considered GRAS.

NEW FOOD TECHNOLOGIES

Food technology is changing rapidly. Scientists continue to research ways to increase crop yields; produce more nutritious foods; grow plants that naturally resist disease, pests, and adverse weather as well as tolerate chemical herbicides; and get rid of bacteria responsible for foodborne illnesses.

Biotechnology

The shelves of just about every American supermarket are lined with foods that have been genetically altered to improve the product's taste, shelf life, or resistance to insects and other pests. Tomatoes, potatoes, squash, corn, and soybeans have been genetically altered through the emerging science of biotechnology. So have ingredients in everything from ketchup and cola to hamburger buns and cake mixes.

Biotechnology enables scientists to modify DNA (deoxyribonucleic acid), the genetic material in living things. Using recombinant DNA methods, scientists identify a desirable gene or several genes in a plant, make copies of those genes, and introduce the gene copies into the genetic code of another plant. The process is called genetic engineering. Usually, the genes are crossed to other crops, allowing rapid development of new varieties.

In 1990 the FDA approved the commercial use of a recombinant DNA-produced enzyme called chymosin (rennet), issuing the first regulation for use of such genetically engineered product. The enzyme rennet, used to help milk clot in making cheese, comes from the lining of calves' stomachs. Scientists copied the gene that produces rennet and reproduced it inside a bacterium. Today, about 50 percent of the rennet used in cheese making is produced through this technique.

In 1992 the FDA announced that food and food ingredients produced by biotechnology are regulated under the federal Food, Drug, and Cosmetic Act of 1938 (52 Stat 1040.) The FDA proposed mandatory rules in January 2001 that would tighten the scrutiny of bioengineered foods. The rules would require that manufacturers of plant-derived, bioengineered foods and animal feeds notify the FDA at least 120 days before the products are marketed.

As part of the notification, the manufacturer would provide information showing that the foods are as safe as their conventional counterparts. Manufacturers have completed voluntary consultations on roughly 50 bioengineered foods using scientific guidelines published by the FDA in 1992. The new proposal would make the current practice of voluntary consultations mandatory and require manufacturers to submit safety and nutritional information to the FDA.

In 1994, for the first time, the FDA approved a whole food derived from a plant modified by biotechnology. The FDA found the fresh tomato Flavr Savr as safe as tomatoes produced by conventional methods. Grocers began selling the Flavr Savr tomato in 1994. The Flavr Savr ripened slower, could remain on the vine longer, and was expected to be of better quality than other tomatoes available in winter.

Experiments are now under way to develop tomatoes that have enhanced levels of lycopene, a plant chemical that gives them their red color. Researchers say lycopene also may offer health benefits due to its apparent antioxidant properties. Antioxidants are thought to neutralize harmful molecules in the human body called "free radicals." These substances, which result from cell metabolism and other causes, may contribute to cancer and cardiovascular disease.

Many genetic modifications have been designed to improve production. About half of the soybeans and about 25 percent of the corn grown in the United States have been bioengineered, according to the USDA. Most of these crop varieties have been designed either to better tolerate herbicides or to resist insects without the need for extensive pesticide spraying. An estimated two-thirds of the processed foods in U.S. supermarkets contain genetically engineered corn, soybeans, or other crops.

Genetically engineered foods that have already been approved, that are awaiting approval, or are being developed include:

- Higher-protein rice.

- Potatoes with higher starch content, which will help reduce the oil absorbed during frying.

- Strawberries with increased ellagic acid, a natural cancer-fighting agent.

- Bananas resistant to fungus.

- Peanuts with improved protein balance.

- Other fruits and vegetables to contain vitamins C and E to protect against heart disease and cancer.

A federally funded study by the National Research Council released in 2000 concluded that there is no evidence that suggests that bioengineered food is unsafe. The study also found that there is no distinction between the health and environmental risks posed by genetically engineered plants and those developed through conventional crossbreeding.

OPPOSITION. The debate over genetically engineered plants began almost as soon as scientists altered plant genes in the early 1980s. Opposition to bioengineered foods has been especially strong in Europe and Japan.

Many consumer and environmental groups believe that genetic engineering is a radical new technology, not an extension of traditional plant breeding. Some of the adverse results that they think are at least theoretically possible with new biotechnology include:

- An increase in levels of naturally occurring toxins and allergens (substances that produce an allergic reaction) or the activation of dormant toxins or allergens.

- A change in the absorption or metabolism of important nutrients.

- A reduction in the effectiveness of some antibiotics through the use of antibiotic-resistant genes.

- Harmful environmental consequences, including negative effects on wildlife and ecosystems.

- A decrease in the quality and nutritional adequacy of animal feed or an increase in the toxins in animal feed.

In September 2000 a consumer group reported that a bioengineered variety of corn not approved for human consumption had been found in taco shells. The corn, dubbed StarLink, was modified to contain a gene from the bacterium *Bacillus thuringiensis* that expressed a protein—Cry9C—toxic to certain insects that endanger the profits of corn growers.

Although StarLink's developer, Aventis, was required to ensure that the bioengineered corn did not go into food, some became mingled with corn destined for human consumption. The presence of an unapproved pesticide in food means that the food is adulterated under the Federal Food, Drug, and Cosmetic Act, enforced by the FDA.

Upon learning of allegations that the taco shells contained StarLink corn, the FDA began a thorough investigation. Kraft Foods, producer of the taco shells, initiated its own investigation and voluntarily recalled millions of taco shells when an independent laboratory found that the shells contained the Cry9C gene. The FDA subsequently confirmed the presence of StarLink in the taco shells.

LABELING. FDA policy dictates that foods derived from biotechnology need not be specially labeled. The FDA will, however, require labeling of genetically engineered food products if the new product differs significantly from its traditional counterpart. For example, labeling would be required if a genetically engineered tomato no longer contained vitamin C. The FDA will also require labeling if a gene from a commonly allergenic food is introduced into a food that was not previously considered allergenic or if the food contains a known toxic substance.

Consumer and environmental groups want the FDA to require premarket testing, a mandatory premarket notification system, and labeling. Some groups that object to genetically engineered foods for moral, ethical, religious, or scientific reasons have threatened legal action against the FDA policy. Critics of the FDA policy insist all genetically engineered foods should be labeled so that consumers can avoid them if they choose. For example, identifying the presence of animal genes in plants may be important for individuals whose diets are restricted for religious reasons. The FDA asserts that in the few cases in which an animal gene might be inserted into a plant, the characteristics of the plant food would not change in a manner relevant to religious beliefs.

Most critics are concerned that the proposed regulations will be inadequate to warn consumers who suffer from allergies when an allergenic protein has been transferred. A study conducted at the University of Nebraska involved feeding subjects modified soybeans injected with a gene from a Brazil nut. Those with an allergy to the nut had an adverse reaction, while those with no allergy were not affected.

Supporters of the FDA policy counter that across-the-board labeling would be expensive and impractical. The components of processed food would be difficult to track, and analytic tests would not always reveal if a food has been genetically engineered. In addition, labels imply a level of risk that is scientifically unsupported and might alarm consumers and jeopardize their acceptance of this technology. Consumer acceptance is key to realizing the potential of new biotechnology.

Novel Macroingredients

Novel macroingredients are typically large quantities of digestible, partially digestible, or nondigestible substances, sometimes 10 percent above the weight of the overall food product. In comparison, food additives are used in amounts below 1 percent by weight. Food producers are developing macroingredients in response to research about the relationship of diet and disease. Their goal is to modify traditional foods so that consumers who want to adhere to diets lower in fat and sugar can achieve this without having to change their eating habits. Olestra is the first macroadditive approved by the FDA.

The government is uncertain how to test the safety of novel macroingredients because there is no precedent for

TABLE 7.3

Some potential uses of Olestra, according to the Proctor & Gamble Company

Snack foods	Restaurant foods
Potato chips[a]	French fries
Corn chips[a]	Fried chicken
Cheese puffs[a]	Fried fish
Crackers[a]	Onion rings
Doughnuts	
Pastries and pies	**Table spreads**
Cakes and cookies	Margarines[b]
Ice cream[b]	Cheeses[b]

Home use
Fried chicken
Grilled meats and vegetables
Sauteed meats and vegetables
Baked desserts and snacks

[a] Use of olestra in savory (salty and spicy) snacks was approved by the FDA on January 24, 1996
[b] Not included in P&G's 1987 petition to the FDA, which excluded uses in table spreads and ice cream

SOURCE: Marion Nestle, "Table 7.5: Some Potential Uses of Olestra, According to the Proctor & Gamble Company," in "The Selling of Olestra," *Public Health Reports*, Vol. 113., no. 6, November/December 1998

evaluating the effects of these products. Conventional methods of animal testing may be inadequate because these ingredients may be chemically more complex than traditional foods and may comprise a greater proportion of the human diet. The usual method for testing toxicity of food additives—giving laboratory animals more than 100 times the likely human intake of the substance—is impractical. Scientists would have to feed laboratory animals quantities they could not physically tolerate. Human testing may be the only way to assess the safety of novel macroingredients. The FDA has not developed a policy or regulations for human clinical trials or determined whether they should be required for novel macroingredients.

OLESTRA. In 1996 the FDA approved olestra, a fat substitute developed by Procter & Gamble, for use in salty and spicy snacks. Although olestra, or sucrose polyester, has properties similar to natural fat, it provides no calories or fat because it is indigestible.

Olestra was approved despite several problems. It absorbs fat-soluble vitamins, such as vitamins A, D, E, and K, from foods eaten at the same time as olestra. It also reduces the absorption of carotenoids—nutrients found in carrots, sweet potatoes, green leafy vegetables, and some animal tissues. Although research on the effects of carotenoids is not conclusive, some studies have shown that they help protect against cancer.

Studies also found that olestra caused severe intestinal cramps, more frequent bowel movements, and diarrhea in some people. The FDA claims these gastrointestinal effects do not have medical consequences

and, in response to these problems, has required that all foods with olestra be labeled with a warning about nutrient loss and possible intestinal distress. Critics, however, charge that Procter & Gamble plans to use olestra in other food items (Table 7.3), which would lead to an increase in olestra consumption.

Marion Nestle, in "The Selling of Olestra" (*Public Health Reports,* Vol. 113, No. 6, November/December 1998), noted that while olestra snacks may be fat free, they are not calorie free. In fact, they reduce by one-half the calories of natural fat products. Nestle believes that just as artificial sweeteners have not lowered overall sugar intake, olestra would probably not reduce the total fat intake.

In March 2001, *Discover Magazine* reported that olestra sales had tumbled from $400,000 in 1998 to $200,000 in 2000 as a result of factors such as the unattractive wording on the label.

Functional Foods

Gingko biloba, St. John's Wort, echinacea, and phosphatidyl serine are just a few dietary supplements found in functional foods—foods that contain a substance or substances that, manufacturers claim, perform a useful function in the body. For example, calcium-fortified orange juice is a functional food that "strengthens the bone." Other functional foods have been touted as capable of increasing energy, preventing depression, boosting the immune system, and increasing mental sharpness. Functional foods are one of the fastest-growing sectors of the food industry, showing annual retail sales of $10 billion. Several large food companies, such as Kellogg and Pillsbury, have produced functional foods in response to the growing demands for them.

In "Functional Foods" (*Nutrition Action Health Letter*, Center for Science in the Public Interest, Washington, D.C., April 1999), Beth Brophy and David Schardt pointed out that it was not until 1993 that the FDA allowed "health claims" on food labels. Prior to this, labels could not claim that foods were capable of preventing a disease. Any reference to a disease meant that the particular food was considered an "unapproved" or illegal drug.

Starting in 1993, Congress told the FDA it could allow a food label to state, for example, that "a diet low in saturated fat and cholesterol can reduce the risk of heart disease," but only if it has the FDA's approval and only if the food isn't unhealthy. Nonetheless, the FDA strictly regulates health claims on food labels and, as of early 1999, had approved only 10 such claims.

In 1994 dietary supplement companies found a loophole in FDA regulations. With the enactment of the Dietary Supplement Health and Education Act (DSHEA; PL 103-417), Congress indicated that there may be a link between dietary supplements and disease prevention, and manufacturers were allowed to claim that a certain supplement can affect the structure or function of the body. For example, the supplement label may claim that it "promotes a healthy heart." Without mention of a disease, such a claim does not require FDA approval.

Large food companies that prepare functional foods are using the same structure and function claims. Some have gone so far as to call their products dietary supplements. In December 1998, McNeil Consumers Healthcare, the U.S. distributor of a Finnish margarine called Benecol, announced that it would sell its product as a dietary supplement.

In May 1999 the FDA approved the sale of Benecol, while announcing that it does not endorse Benecol or its claims. The FDA had simply reviewed the testing done by McNeil and told the company it would not violate FDA labeling regulations if the product label states Benecol contains an ingredient that "helps promote healthy cholesterol levels."

Brophy and Schardt are concerned that, unlike food additives or drugs, ingredients in functional foods are not required to undergo premarket evaluations to determine if they might cause serious conditions, such as cancer or liver toxicity. Some individuals have been known to develop severe allergies to dietary supplements, the health-claim components of functional foods. Still others have suffered adverse reactions from mixtures of medicine and dietary supplements.

Irradiation

The term irradiation refers to the exposure of food to radiation in order to eliminate bacteria. In 1963 irradiation was first approved by the FDA for wheat and wheat flour. Since then the FDA has approved irradiation for spices and seasonings, enzymes, fruits, vegetables, grain products, and poultry. In December 1997 the FDA concluded that irradiation is safe for raw meat. However, since the USDA regulates the processing and labeling of red meat, irradiation will not be authorized until the USDA completes writing the implementation regulations.

According to FDA scientists, irradiation eliminates or decreases bacterial pathogens, insects, and parasites. It diminishes spoilage and, in some fruits and vegetables, prevents sprouting and delays the ripening process. They claim the process is safe and does not remove nutrients from the food or make it radioactive. It also will not noticeably change food taste, texture, or appearance.

More than 40 countries—including Canada, France, China, Japan, Italy, Russia, and Mexico—have been using food irradiation since the 1960s. American astronauts have eaten irradiated foods since 1972, and such professional organizations as the American Medical Association and the American Dietetic Association have endorsed irra-

TABLE 7.4

Estimated annual quantities and percentage of consumption for irradiated food, as of January 2000

Food product	Amount irradiated (millions of pounds)	Percentage of annual consumption
Spices and dry or dehydrated aromatic vegetable substances	95.0	9.5
Fruits and vegetables	1.5	0.002
Fresh and frozen uncooked poultry	0.5	0.002
Total	**97.0**	

Notes: Refrigerated and frozen uncooked beef, pork, lamb, and goat have been approved for irradiation; however, as of January 2000, these products were not available commercially.

SOURCE: "Estimated Annual Quantities and Percentage of Consumption for Irradiated Food in the United States, as of January 2000" in *Food Irradiation: Available Research Indicates that Benefits Outweigh Risks,* U.S. General Accounting Office, Washington, D.C., 2000

diation. However, not everyone approves of exposing food to radiant energy. Opponents are concerned that irradiation facilities could threaten worker safety and public health. Some believe that irradiation may result in carcinogenic (cancer-causing) food.

As of early 2000 the majority of irradiated foods consumed in the U.S. was in the category of spices or other dried vegetable substances, accounting for 95 of the 97 million pounds of irradiated food product. (See Table 7.4.)

PESTICIDES

Regulatory Monitoring

Three federal agencies share responsibility in regulating pesticides. The FDA is charged with enforcing pesticide residue tolerances and ensuring that environmental contaminants in food and animal feed are within safe levels. (Residue tolerance refers to the maximum amount of a pesticide residue that is permitted in or on a food). The Environmental Protection Agency (EPA) is responsible for registering the use of pesticides after ensuring that their use will not cause an unreasonable risk. The EPA also establishes the legal maximum level of pesticide residues allowed in each specific food. In addition, the EPA obtains information on industrial chemical effects that present unreasonable risks to people and the environment, and controls their production, distribution, and disposal. The third agency, the USDA, is responsible for regulating pesticides in meat, poultry, and egg products.

FDA DOMESTIC MONITORING. In *Food and Drug Administration Pesticide Program—Residue Monitoring 1999* (Washington, D.C., 1999), the FDA analyzed 3,426 food samples from 47 states (no samples were collected from New Hampshire, Rhode Island, and Oklahoma) and Puerto Rico. Nearly two-thirds (60.2 percent) had no

FIGURE 7.1

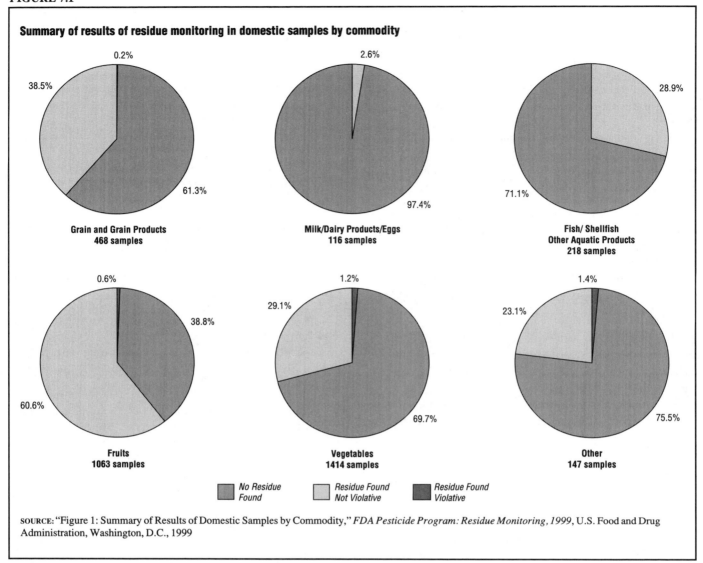

Summary of results of residue monitoring in domestic samples by commodity

Grain and Grain Products
468 samples

Milk/Dairy Products/Eggs
116 samples

Fish/ Shellfish
Other Aquatic Products
218 samples

Fruits
1063 samples

Vegetables
1414 samples

Other
147 samples

No Residue Found   Residue Found Not Violative   Residue Found Violative

SOURCE: "Figure 1: Summary of Results of Domestic Samples by Commodity," *FDA Pesticide Program: Residue Monitoring, 1999*, U.S. Food and Drug Administration, Washington, D.C., 1999

detectable pesticide residues and only 0.8 percent had violative residues. The FDA defines a violative residue as "a residue that exceeds a tolerance or a residue at a level of regulatory significance for which no tolerance has been established in the sampled food." Figure 7.1 shows the proportions of the domestic samples by commodity group with no residues found, nonviolative residues found, and violative residues found.

The FDA's Total Diet Study, conducted in 1999, is different from regulatory monitoring in that it determined pesticide residues in 1,040 food items prepared for consumption. As Table 7.5 indicates, the pesticide residues shown were found in more than 2 percent of samples. The five most frequently occurring residues have been the same for several years. All, however, are below regulatory limits.

FDA IMPORT MONITORING. In 1999 the FDA also analyzed food samples from 94 countries. Mexico was the source of the largest number of samples, reflecting the

volume and diversity of commodities imported from that country. Of the 6,012 samples analyzed, 65 percent had no pesticide residues detected, and 3.1 percent had violative residues. (See Figure 7.2.)

Problems with Monitoring Pesticides in Imports

The United States has no jurisdiction over food producers in other countries. Consequently, the federal agencies must rely on the foreign countries' food safety systems and/or U.S. inspection at the port of entry. The U.S. General Accounting Office (GAO) has repeatedly reported to Congress that this is a flawed food safety system, but nothing has been done to correct it.

While the USDA has the power to require that an exporting country's meat inspection system meet American standards before that country can ship products to the United States, the FDA has no such power. The FDA must rely on exporting countries to voluntarily comply with

U.S. food standards. In addition, produce importers retain possession of their shipments during investigation of suspected unsafe food and can distribute them for sale while the FDA conducts pesticide residue testing. Consequently, perishable fruits and vegetables may be sold and consumed before the results of testing are available.

Children Are Vulnerable to Pesticides

Children are at greater risk of harm from pesticides than are adults. Relative to their size, they eat more than adults do, and their bodies are still developing.

Richard Wiles and colleagues, in *How 'Bout Them Apples?: Pesticides in Children's Food Ten Years After Alar* (Environmental Working Group, Washington, D.C., 1999), reported that each day, over 610,000 children one to five years old ingest an unsafe dose of neurotoxic pesticides. In addition, 61,000 of these children exceed 10 times the EPA "safe" dose for pesticides. (See Table 7.6.)

The Environmental Working Group (EWG) claims that 10 years after the pesticide alar was pulled off the market due to public outrage, apples continue to be loaded with pesticides. More than one-half of the 610,500 children exposed to unsafe insecticides get that dose by eating an apple or an apple product. Over 80 percent of children ages one to five who are exposed to 10 times the daily EPA "safe" dose of pesticides get that dose from eating peaches, apples, and grapes (See Table 7.7.)

The EWG recommends that parents feed their children fruits and vegetables with consistently low pesticide residues. (See Table 7.8.)

Regulation Affecting Cancer-Causing Pesticide Residues

In 1996 Congress passed legislation changing the requirements for cancer-causing ingredients in foods. The Delaney Clause, passed in 1958, banned any cancer-causing residues in processed foods. The new provisions (part of the Food Protection Act, PL 104-170) would allow pesticide residues only if there is a "reasonable certainty" that they would cause no harm. "Reasonable certainty" has been defined as a lifetime risk of developing cancer of no more than one in 1 million. Special attention would be required to ensure that no harm would result to infants and children from cumulative effects. The legislation applies equally to raw and processed foods. One of the reasons for the change is that scientists are now able to detect residues in amounts far lower than they once could.

ORGANIC FOODS

The word "organic" usually means the food has been grown without synthetic pesticides and/or fertilizers. In 1990 the Organic Foods Production Act (PL 101-624) mandated that the USDA develop national standards and a

TABLE 7.5

Frequency of occurrence of pesticide residues found in total diet study foods in 1999[a]

Pesticide[b]	Total No. of Findings	Occurrence, %
DDT	225	22
chlorpyrifos-methyl	188	18
malathion	175	17
endosulfan	151	15
dieldrin	145	14
chlorpyrifos	93	9
chlorpropham	70	7
permethrin	54	5
iprodione	48	5
chlordane	36	3
heptachlor	36	3
lindane	33	3
thiabendazole[c]	33	3
BHC, alpha+beta+delta	32	3
hexachlorobenzene	32	3
carbaryl[d]	31	3
methamidophos	29	3
methoxychlor	29	3
dicloran	28	3
dimethoate	24	2

[a] Based on 4 market baskets analyzed in 1999 consisting of 260 items each (1040 total). Only those found in >2% of the samples are shown.
[b] Isomers, metabolites, and related compounds are included with the "parent" pesticide from which they arise.
[c] Reflects overall incidence; however, only 67 selected foods per market basket (*i.e.*, 268 items total) were analyzed for the benzimidazole fungicides thiabendazole and benomyl.
[d] Reflects overall incidence; however, only 96 selected foods per market basket (*i.e.*, 384 items total) were analyzed for N- methylcarbamates.

SOURCE: "Table 6: Frequency of Occurrence of Pesticide Residues Found in Total Diet Study Foods in 1999," *FDA Pesticide Program: Residue Monitoring, 1999*, U.S. Food and Drug Administration, Washington, D.C., 1999

TABLE 7.6

Children aged 1-5 who get an unsafe dose of neurotoxic pesticides in food each day, 1989–98

Age	Estimated number of children exceeding the EPA "safe" dose per day	Percent of population	Children exceeding 10 times the EPA "safe" dose per day
1	137,200	3.4%	13,500
2	131,400	3.3%	13,500
3	130,000	3.2%	13,900
4	104,300	2.6%	9,700
5	107,600	2.7%	10,400
Total	**610,400**	**3.1%**	**61,000**

Figures rounded to nearest hundred.
Compiled from USDA food consumption data 1989–1996, USDA and FDA pesticide residue data 1991–1997, and U.S. EPA 1998 data.

SOURCE: Richard Wiles, Kenneth Cook, Todd Hettenbach, and Christopher Campbell, "Table 1: More than 600,000 children under age six get an unsafe dose of neurotoxic pesticides in food each day," in *How 'Bout Them Apples? Pesticides in Children's Food Ten Years After,* Environmental Working Group, Washington, D.C., 1999

certification program for organically grown agricultural products, and in December 1997 the USDA proposed a national standard for the production, handling, and processing of organically grown agricultural products.

FIGURE 7.2

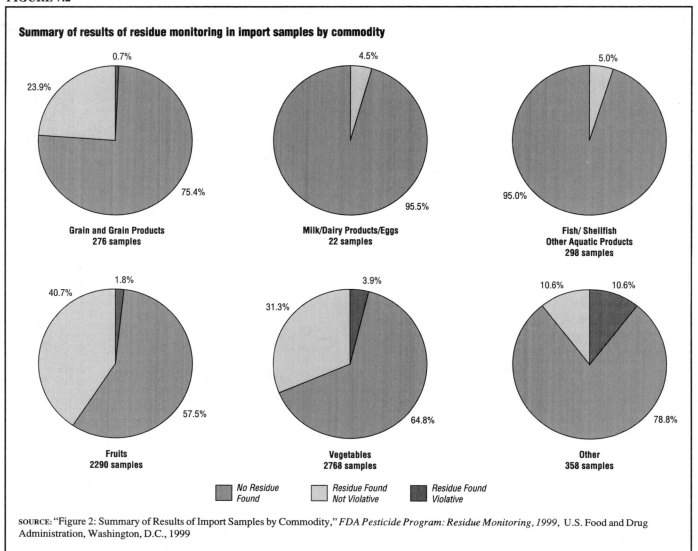

Summary of results of residue monitoring in import samples by commodity

Grain and Grain Products
276 samples
0.7% / 23.9% / 75.4%

Milk/Dairy Products/Eggs
22 samples
4.5% / 95.5%

Fish/ Shellfish
Other Aquatic Products
298 samples
5.0% / 95.0%

Fruits
2290 samples
1.8% / 40.7% / 57.5%

Vegetables
2768 samples
3.9% / 31.3% / 64.8%

Other
358 samples
10.6% / 10.6% / 78.8%

No Residue Found | Residue Found Not Violative | Residue Found Violative

SOURCE: "Figure 2: Summary of Results of Import Samples by Commodity," *FDA Pesticide Program: Residue Monitoring, 1999,* U.S. Food and Drug Administration, Washington, D.C., 1999

TABLE 7.7

Estimated number of children exposed to 10 times the EPA "safe" dose per day

Food	1-year-olds	2-year-olds	3-year-olds	4-year-olds	5-year-olds	Total
Peaches	5,700	4,500	5,700	2,800	3,500	22,100
Apples	2,600	4,300	4,100	3,700	3,200	18,000
Grapes	2,100	2,400	2,200	1,700	1,700	10,200
Nectarines	500	600	800	300	700	2,800
Pears	600	700	400	400	400	2,600
Fresh green beans	400	300	300	300	300	1,600
Total for all foods	**13,200**	**13,300**	**13,700**	**9,500**	**10,200**	**59,900**

SOURCE: Richard Wiles, Kenneth Cook, Todd Hettenbach, and Christopher Campbell, "Estimated number of children exposed to 10 times the EPA 'safe' dose/day from individual foods," in *How 'Bout Them Apples? Pesticides in Children's Food Ten Years After,* Environmental Working Group, Washington, D.C., 1999

Essentially, the new organic standard offers a national definition for the term "organic." It details the methods, practices, and substances that can be used in producing and handling organic crops and livestock, as well as processed products. It established clear organic labeling criteria, and specifically prohibits the use of genetic engineering methods, ionizing radiation, and sewage sludge for fertilization.

All agricultural products labeled organic must originate from farms or handling operations certified by a

TABLE 7.8

Ten foods most contaminated by pesticides and ten least contaminated foods, 1992–97

Most Contaminated Foods		Least Contaminated Foods	
Rank	Food	Rank	Food
1	Apples	1	Corn
2	Spinach	2	Cauliflower
3	Peaches	3	Sweet Peas
4	Pears	4	Asparagus
5	Strawberries	5	Broccoli
6	Grapes - Chile	6	Pineapple
7	Potatoes	7	Onions
8	Red Raspberries	8	Bananas
9	Celery	9	Watermelon
10	Green Beans	10	Cherries - Chile

Compiled from USDA and FDA pesticide residue data 1992–1997.

SOURCE: Richard Wiles, Kenneth Cook, Todd Hettenbach, and Christopher Campbell, "Table 3: Parents can reduce health risks to their children by feeding them fruits and vegetables with consistently low pesticide residues," in *How 'Bout Them Apples? Pesticides in Children's Food Ten Years After*, Environmental Working Group, Washington, D.C., 1999

FIGURE 7.3

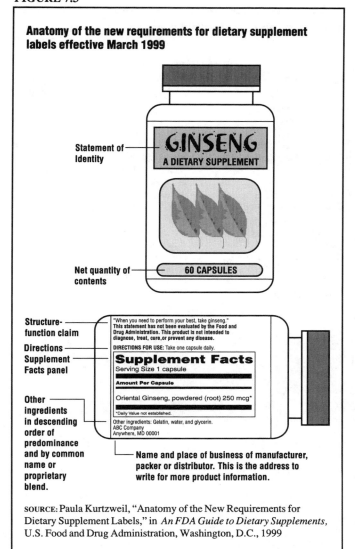

Anatomy of the new requirements for dietary supplement labels effective March 1999

SOURCE: Paula Kurtzweil, "Anatomy of the New Requirements for Dietary Supplement Labels," in *An FDA Guide to Dietary Supplements*, U.S. Food and Drug Administration, Washington, D.C., 1999

state or private agency accredited by the USDA. Farms and handling operations that sell less than $5,000 worth per year of organic agricultural products are exempt from certification.

New organic labeling on products are expected to be fully implemented by mid-2002.

Because organic farming is labor-intensive and done on a relatively small scale, (accounting for only 1.2 percent of U.S. food sales), organic products cost more than other foods, sometimes as high as 50 percent more. Nonetheless, organic farming has become a $4 billion business, increasing about 20 percent annually since 1990. The industry is supported by people who want healthy food free of chemicals.

It is important to remember that the label "certified organic" is not a nutrition claim. Organic foods do not contain more or different nutrients than regular food. Furthermore, while organic foods are produced without the use of artificial chemicals, the possibility remains that they were exposed to residual chemicals in the environment, or disease-carrying bacteria. So a certified organic label is not a guarantee of safety, either. Still, any organic products should have been exposed to far fewer chemicals and other high-technology treatments than non-organic foods typically are. For many people this is reason enough to eat organic food.

DIETARY SUPPLEMENTS

Definition of Dietary Supplements

For many years the FDA regulated dietary supplements as food, considering them to consist of essential nutrients, such as proteins, vitamins, and minerals. In 1990 the Nutrition Labeling and Education Act (PL 101-

535) included "herbs, or similar nutritional substances" under the category of dietary supplements. In 1994, as a result of vigorous lobbying by the dietary supplement industry, Congress indicated that there might be a link between dietary supplements and disease prevention. Under the Dietary Supplement and Health Education Act (DSHEA; PL 103-417), Congress added items such as ginseng, fish oils, psyllium (a seed used as a mild laxative), enzymes, and mixtures of any of these ingredients to their definition of dietary supplements.

Unlike prescription and over-the-counter drugs, dietary supplements are not required to undergo evaluations for safety or effectiveness before they are sent to market. The DSHEA allows dietary supplement manufacturers to make almost any claim for their products as long as they print the disclaimer on the label that the products "have not been evaluated by the Food and Drug Administration." After the passage of DSHEA, dietary supplement sales climbed from $8 billion in 1994 to $12 billion in 1997.

TABLE 7.9

Supplements associated with illnesses and injuries, 1998

NAME	POSSIBLE HEALTH HAZARDS
Herbal Ingredients	
Chaparral (a traditional American Indian medicine)	liver disease, possibly irreversible
Comfrey	obstruction of blood flow to liver, possibly leading to death
Slimming/dieter's teas	nausea, diarrhea, vomiting, stomach cramps, chronic constipation, fainting, possibly death
Ephedra (also known as Ma huang, Chinese Ephedra and epitonin)	ranges from high blood pressure, irregular heartbeat, nerve damage, injury, insomnia, tremors, and headaches to seizures, heart attack, stroke, and death
Germander	liver disease, possibly leading to death
Lobelia (also known as Indian tobacco)	range from breathing problems at low doses to sweating, rapid heartbeat, low blood pressure, and possibly coma and death at higher doses
Magnolia-Stephania preparation	kidney disease, possibly leading to permanent kidney failure
Willow bark	Reye syndrome, a potentially fatal disease associated with aspirin intake in children with chickenpox or flu symptoms; allergic reaction in adults. (Willow bark is marketed as an aspirin-free product, although it actually contains an ingredient that converts to the same active ingredient in aspirin.)
Wormwood	neurological symptoms, characterized by numbness of legs and arms, loss of intellect, delirium, and paralysis
Vitamins and Essential Minerals	
Vitamin A in doses of 25,000 or more International Units a day	birth defects, bone abnormalities, and severe liver disease
Vitamin B₆ in doses above 100 milligrams a day	balance difficulties, nerve injury causing changes in touch sensation
Niacin in slow-released doses of 500 mg or more a day or immediate-release doses of 750 mg or more a day	range from stomach pain, vomiting, bloating, nausea, cramping, and diarrhea to liver disease, muscle disease, eye damage, and heart injury
Selenium in doses of about 800 micrograms to 1,000 mcg a day	tissue damage
Other Supplements	
Germanium (a nonessential mineral)	kidney damage, possibly death
L-tryptophan (an amino acid)	eosinophilia myalgia syndrome, a potentially fatal blood disorder that can cause high fever, muscle and joint pain, weakness, skin rash, and swelling of the arms and legs

SOURCE: "An FDA Guide to Dietary Supplements," *FDA Consumer,* U.S. Federal Drug Administration, Washington, D.C., 1998

New FDA Regulation for Dietary Supplements

Effective March 23, 1999, the FDA required that dietary supplement labels include a Supplement Facts panel, patterned after the Nutrition Facts panel on food items. According to the FDA, labels must identify dietary supplements as such. Products with botanical ingredients must identify the part of the plant used. Supplements labeled "high potency" and "antioxidant" must also meet FDA criteria. (See Figure 7.3.)

FIGURE 7.4

Where shoppers think food safety problems are most likely to occur

Food processors/manufacturers	27%
Restaurants	24%
At home	14%
During transportation	8%
Grocery stores	7%
Other	7%
All	5%
On farms	2%

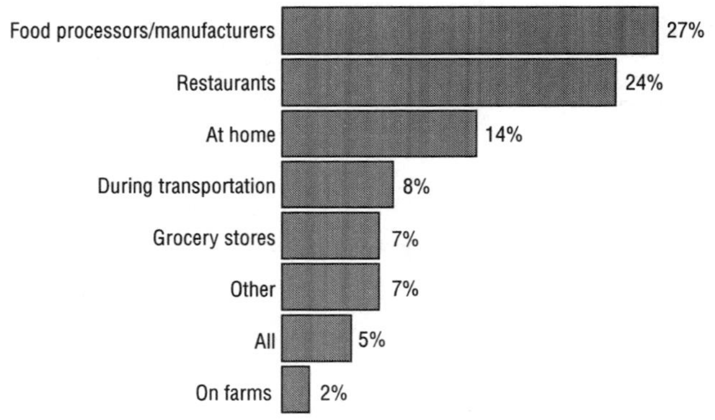

SOURCE: "Figure 18: Where Shoppers Think Food Safety Problems Are Most Likely to Occur," in *Trends in the United States: Consumer Attitudes & the Supermarket 2000,* Food Marketing Institute, Washington, D.C., 2000

Some Dietary Supplements Are Dangerous

In 1998 the *New England Journal of Medicine (NEJM)* reported a number of adverse effects among individuals using dietary supplements. Some persons take supplements to heal ailments. Robert S. DiPaola and colleagues, in "Clinical and Biologic Activity of an Estrogenic Herbal Combination (PC-SPES) in Prostate Cancer" (*NEJM,* Vol. 339, No. 12, September 17, 1998), found that PC-SPES, an unregulated combination of eight herbs, produced unexpected effects similar to that of estrogen.

Richard J. Ko of the California Department of Health Services, in "Adulterants in Asian Patent Medicines" (*NEJM,* Vol. 339, No. 12, September 17, 1998), reported that toxic levels of metals, such as lead, arsenic, and mercury, have been found in Asian patent medicines collected from California retail herbal stores. Chemicals, such as ephedrine, were also common components not declared on the supplement label.

Many cases of immediate adverse reactions to dietary supplements have also been reported. Kava has been known to cause drowsiness, and echinacea has brought on allergic reactions. According to the FDA, since 1993, the herbal stimulant Ma-huang, or Chinese ephedra, has caused at least 30 deaths and more than 800 cases of adverse side effects, including strokes, heart attacks, seizures, and high blood pressure. Ephedra, an amphetamine-like compound, exerts powerful stimulant effects on the nervous system and heart. So-called herbal fen-phen products, which consumers may associate with the diet drugs recently withdrawn by the FDA, contain ephedra as their main ingredient. Table 7.9 shows dietary supplements that have been associated with illnesses and injuries.

TABLE 7.10

Likelihood of purchasing products modified by biotechnology to taste better or fresher, 1996 and 2000

Question: All things being equal, how likely would you be to buy a new variety of produce, like a tomato or potato, if it had been modified by "biotechnology" to taste better or fresher?

| | Jan. 2000 Base | Very or Somewhat Likely | | Jan. 2000 | | | |
		Jan. 1996 %	Jan. 2000 %	Very Likely %	Somewhat Likely %	Not Too Likely %	Not at All Likely %
Total	**1,000**	**58**	**54**	**16**	**38**	**23**	**20**
Gender							
Men	262	67	55	19	36	22	18
Women	738	53	52	14	38	23	20
Work 20+ hrs/wk	391	52	53	12	41	26	19
Work 0–19 hrs/wk	324	55	54	17	37	19	22
Type of Household							
With children	367	54	51	13	38	26	19
Aged 0–6	181	54	48	14	34	31	17
Aged 7–17	272	55	52	12	40	24	21
No children	608	60	55	17	38	21	20
Size of Household							
One	173	69	59	20	39	18	17
Two	339	56	53	14	39	22	22
Three–four	330	55	54	16	38	23	18
Five or more	132	59	51	14	37	27	20
Income							
$15,000 or less	104	54	55	17	38	17	20
$15,001–$25,000	109	63	58	19	39	23	17
$25,001–$35,000	151	56	54	16	38	24	18
$35,001–$50,000	172	57	56	15	41	22	19
$50,001–$75,000	159	63	53	17	36	26	17
$75,001 or more	125	61	50	16	34	30	14
Education							
High school or less	411	58	55	15	40	18	23
Some college or more	557	58	52	16	36	26	18

May not add to 100 percent due to rounding.

SOURCE: "Table 48: Likelihood to Buy Products Modified by Biotechnology to Taste Better/Fresher," in *Trends in the United States: Consumer Attitudes & the Supermarket 2000,* Food Marketing Institute, Washington, D.C., 2000

PUBLIC OPINION

Food Safety Information and Concerns

Nutrition and product safety ranked second only to taste when consumers were asked what factors were important when they shopped for food. In the 2000 Food Marketing Institute survey *Trends in the United States—Consumer Attitudes and the Supermarket 2000*, 71 percent of shoppers rated product safety as very important, and 91 percent rated safety as very or somewhat important. Nearly three-quarters of consumers were confident that the food in their supermarket was safe. Shoppers in the East were less confident—probably due to an outbreak of *E. coli* food poisoning at a New York county fair a few months prior to the survey.

Consumers believed that food safety problems could occur at various points in the food distribution chain, from the farm to the home. Shoppers thought that food processors (27 percent) and restaurants (24 percent) were the points most likely to experience problems. Third most likely was the home, according to 14 percent of shoppers. Only 7 percent of respondents felt that supermarkets were likely to experience food safety problems. (See Figure 7.4.)

FIGURE 7.5

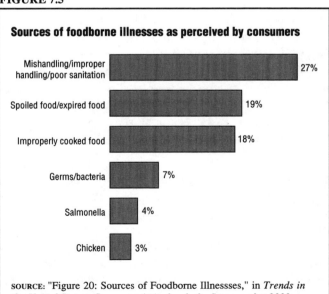

Sources of foodborne illnesses as perceived by consumers

SOURCE: "Figure 20: Sources of Foodborne Illnessses," in *Trends in the United States: Consumer Attitudes & the Supermarket 2000,* Food Marketing Institute, Washington, D.C., 2000

TABLE 7.11

Likelihood of purchasing products modified by biotechnology to resist insect damage and require fewer pesticide applications, 1996 and 2000

Question: All things being equal, how likely would you be to buy a new variety of produce if it had been modified by "biotechnology" to resist insect damage and require fewer pesticide applications?

| | Jan. 2000 Base | Very or Somewhat Likely | | Jan. 2000 | | | |
		Jan. 1996 %	Jan. 2000 %	Very Likely %	Somewhat Likely %	Not Too Likely %	Not at all Likely %
Total	**1,000**	**77**	**63**	**26**	**37**	**16**	**17**
Gender							
Men	262	82	66	27	39	16	16
Women	738	75	61	25	36	17	17
Work 20+ hrs/wk	391	77	65	23	42	17	14
Work 0–19 hrs/wk	324	73	58	29	29	16	20
Type of Household							
With children	367	77	66	25	41	15	16
Aged 0–6	181	79	68	25	43	14	13
Aged 7–17	272	76	65	26	39	15	17
No children	608	77	62	27	35	17	17
Size of Household							
One	173	78	61	25	36	15	18
Two	339	77	60	26	34	18	19
Three–four	330	77	65	27	38	17	14
Five or more	132	78	69	27	42	12	15
Income							
$15,000 or less	104	62	62	26	36	11	22
$15,001–$25,000	109	75	59	26	33	19	18
$25,001–$35,000	151	76	66	28	38	16	13
$35,001–$50,000	172	85	66	27	39	17	15
$50,001–$75,000	159	77	63	23	40	19	11
$75,001 or more	125	91	71	26	45	11	13
Education							
High school or less	411	49	59	27	32	14	21
Some college or less	557	48	65	25	40	18	13

May not add to 100 percent due to rounding.

SOURCE: "Table 49: Likelihood to Buy Products Modified by Biotechnology to Resist Insect Damage and Require Fewer Pesticide Applications," in *Trends in the United States: Consumer Attitudes & the Supermarket 2000,* Food Marketing Institute, Washington, D.C., 2000

Shoppers Aware of Foodborne Illness Risk

While shoppers recognized the dangers of mishandling food, there was a significant decrease in those who reported that it was very or fairly common for people to become ill because of the way food was handled or prepared in their homes. In 2000 less than one-third of shoppers thought this was very or fairly common compared with 41 percent in 1999.

Respondents felt that the most common sources of food poisoning were mishandling, spoiled food, and improperly cooked foods. Responses were similar to 1999, with 27 percent citing mishandling or poor sanitation as the most common source, followed by spoiled food (19 percent) and improperly cooked foods (18 percent). (See Figure 7.5.) Respondents also cited germs, *Salmonella*, and lack of refrigeration as culprits in causing food poisoning.

Shoppers were aware of proper food handling to keep food safe. They mentioned a number of things they did in their own kitchens. Many of these food handling practices were publicized in the Fight Bac! Campaign, sponsored by the Partnership for Food Safety Education, a national organization dedicated to informing consumers about the importance of food safety. The action most frequently mentioned was washing hands and surfaces, followed by washing vegetables and cleaning food, cooking properly, and refrigerating foods promptly.

Attitudes Toward Biotechnology

The Food Marketing Institute also asked consumers about their likelihood to buy a new variety of produce if it had been modified by biotechnology to taste better. Approximately one-half (54 percent) of respondents were very or somewhat likely, down from 58 percent in 1996. (See Table 7.10.)

Consumers were more willing to buy biotechnology-modified products if it meant resistance to insect damage and fewer required pesticide applications. Nearly two-thirds (63 percent) of respondents were very or somewhat likely, though this was down from 77 percent in 1996. (See Table 7.11.)

CHAPTER 8
PERCEPTION AND REALITY IN AMERICAN DIETS

Nearly all Americans have received information about the health benefits of lowering cholesterol intake, cutting back on fat, and eating more fruits and vegetables, but has this led to people changing their eating habits? While many are aware of the importance of a healthful diet, they are often confused by conflicting messages from the health and food industries. Others, while they might know what a healthful diet is, put convenience and taste ahead of healthful eating.

A survey by the National Cancer Institute, a branch of the National Institutes of Health, found that the average American eats only about three servings of fruits and vegetables a day. Forty-two percent eat less than two servings a day. Considering that the *Dietary Guidelines for Americans* recommends five to nine servings of fruits and vegetables daily, most Americans still have a way to go. Another indication that Americans have not improved their eating habits, despite greater knowledge of the nutri-

TABLE 8.1

Food group servings perceived, consumed, and recommended by gender/age group, 2000

	Grains	Fruits	Vegetables	Milk	Meat, etc.	Other (fats, oils, and sweets)
Females 19-24						
Perceived	3.2	2.6	2.6	3.2	3.5	2.2
Consumed	4.2	0.8	1.7	1.2	1.6	3.0
Recommended	9	3	4	2	2.4	Use sparingly
Females 25-50						
Perceived	2.9	2.2	2.5	2.3	3.0	2.1
Consumed	4.6	0.8	2.0	1.0	1.7	3.2
Recommended	9	3	4	2	2.4	Use sparingly
Females 51 +						
Perceived	2.5	2.4	2.6	2.1	2.7	1.6
Consumed	4.7	1.5	2.2	1.0	1.7	3.1
Recommended	7.4	2.5	3.5	3	2.2	Use sparingly
Males19-24						
Perceived	2.9	2.1	2.2	3.1	3.7	2.1
Consumed	5.5	0.6	2.3	1.6	2.3	4.1
Recommended	11	4	5	2	2.8	Use sparingly
Males 25-50						
Perceived	2.9	2.2	2.4	2.2	3.4	2.1
Consumed	5.9	0.9	2.5	1.2	2.5	4.0
Recommended	11	4	5	2	2.8	Use sparingly
Males 51 +						
Perceived	2.7	2.2	2.5	2.1	3.1	1.7
Consumed	6.2	1.3	2.7	1.1	2.4	4.5
Recommended	9.1	3.2	4.2	3	2.5	Use sparingly

Recommended servings based on energy RDA for gender/age groups.

SOURCE: *Consumption of Food Group Servings: People's Perceptions vs. Reality,* Nutrition Insights 20, U.S. Department of Agriculture, Center for Nutrition Policy and Promotion, Washington, D.C., 2000

TABLE 8.2

Recommended number of servings per day for age/gender categories

Age/gender category	Kilocalories	Grains	Vegetables	Fruits	Milk	Meat
Children 1-3	1,300	6.0[a]	3.0[a]	2.0[a]	2.0[a]	2.0[a]
*	1,600	6.0	3.0	2.0	2.0	2.0
Children 4-6	1,800	7.0	3.3	2.3	2.0	2.1
Females 51+	1,900	7.4	3.5	2.5	2.0	2.2
Children 7-10	2,000	7.8	3.7	2.7	2.0	2.3
Females 11-50	2,200	9.0	4.0	3.0	2.0	2.4
Males 51+	2,300	9.1	4.2	3.2	2.0	2.5
Males 11-14	2,500	9.9	4.5	3.5	3.0	2.6
*	2,800	11.0	5.0	4.0	2.0	2.8
Males 19-50	2,900	11.0	5.0	4.0	2.0[b]	2.8
Males 15-18	3,000	11.0	5.0	4.0	2.0	2.8

[a] Portion sizes are reduced for children age 1-3.
[b] Is 3 servings for persons age 11 to 24.
*RDA levels included in the Food Guide Pyramid.

SOURCE: Jayachandran Variyam, James Blaylock, David Smallwood, and Peter Basiotis, "Table 2: Recommended number of servings per day for age/gender categories," in *USDA's Healthy Eating Index and Nutrition Information,* Technical Bulletin No. 1866, U.S. Department of Agriculture, Economic Research Service, Washington, D.C., 1998

FIGURE 8.1

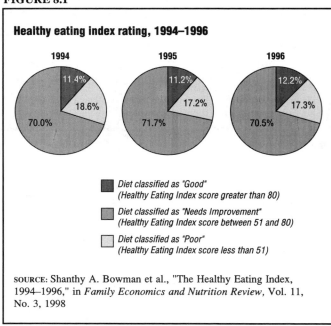

Healthy eating index rating, 1994–1996

1994 / 1995 / 1996

- Diet classified as "Good" (Healthy Eating Index score greater than 80)
- Diet classified as "Needs Improvement" (Healthy Eating Index score between 51 and 80)
- Diet classified as "Poor" (Healthy Eating Index score less than 51)

SOURCE: Shanthy A. Bowman et al., "The Healthy Eating Index, 1994–1996," in *Family Economics and Nutrition Review,* Vol. 11, No. 3, 1998

TABLE 8.3

Americans' interest in improving their diet, by selected characteristics and nutrition-related beliefs, 1991–94

	Interest in improving the diet		
	Yes	No[1]	Needs no improvement
Sample	409	590	852
Percent	23	37	40
		Percent	
Race			
White	80	93	92
Non-white	20	7	8
Gender			
Male	37	62	53
Female	63	38	47
Percent of Poverty			
130 and under	36	24	22
131 and over	64	76	78
Beliefs			
Diet is unhealthful.	58	32	5
Too much emphasis is placed on nutrition.	37	69	48
Eating healthfully is too complicated.	70	69	40
Most snacks consumed are unhealthful.	77	68	49

[1] Not interested in improving the diet or believes changing the diet will do no good.

SOURCE: "Table 1. Americans' interest in improving their diet, by selected characteristics and nutrition-related beliefs, 1991–94," in *Beliefs and Attitudes of Americans Toward their Diet,* Nutrition Insights 19, U.S. Department of Agriculture, Center for Nutrition Policy and Promotion, Washington, D.C., 2000

tional benefits of a healthful diet, is the growing proportion of overweight American adults and children.

PERCEIVED INTAKE VERSUS ACTUAL CONSUMPTION

P. P. Basiotis, Mark Lino, and Julia Dinkins ("Consumption of Food Group Servings: People's Perception vs. Reality," *Nutrition Insights,* USDA, October 2000) compared the number of food group servings that people estimate consuming with the number of servings from records they kept over a two-week period. As Table 8.1 indicates, all gender and age groups perceived consuming fewer

grain servings (2.5 to 3.2) daily than what they actually ate (4.2 to 6.2 servings). Although their consumption of grains per day was above what they believed, it was still below the Pyramid recommendations. For example, females ages

FIGURE 8.2

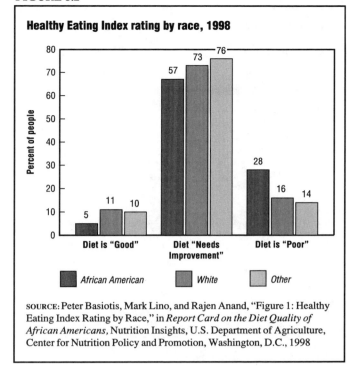

Healthy Eating Index rating by race, 1998

SOURCE: Peter Basiotis, Mark Lino, and Rajen Anand, "Figure 1: Healthy Eating Index Rating by Race," in *Report Card on the Diet Quality of African Americans,* Nutrition Insights, U.S. Department of Agriculture, Center for Nutrition Policy and Promotion, Washington, D.C., 1998

TABLE 8.4

Knowledge of nutrient content in U.S. households, 1989–90

Question	Correct	Incorrect
	Percent	
Which has more fiber?		
Fruit or meat	77.7	22.3
Cornflakes or oatmeal	79.5	20.5
Whole-wheat bread or white bread	91.8	8.2
Orange juice or an apple	74.0	26.0
Kidney beans or lettuce	56.3	43.7
Popcorn or pretzels	73.6	26.4
Which has more cholesterol?		
Liver or T-bone steak	52.3	47.7
Butter or margarine	87.2	12.8
Egg whites or yolks	84.6	15.4
Skim milk or whole milk	95.0	5.0
Which has more fat?		
Regular hamburger or ground round	87.8	12.2
Loin pork chops or spare ribs	72.0	28.0
Hot dogs or ham	61.3	38.7
Peanuts or popcorn	90.5	9.5
Yogurt or sour cream	85.9	14.1
Porterhouse steak or round steak	58.8	41.2
Ice cream or sherbet	95.0	5.0
Roast chicken leg or fried chicken leg	94.6	5.4
Which kind of fat (saturated, polyunsaturated) is more likely to be a liquid rather than a solid? Or are they equally likely to be liquids?	29.6	70.4
Is cholesterol found in vegetables and vegetable oils, animal products, or all foods containing fat or oil?	38.7	61.3
If a food is labeled cholesterol-free, is it also low in saturated fat, high in saturated fat, or either?	55.6	44.4

Note: Based on the 1989–90 Diet Health Knowledge Survey.

SOURCE: Jayachandran Variyam, James Blaylock, David Smallwood, and Peter Basiotis, "Table 3: Nutrient content knowledge questions and percent responses," in *USDA's Healthy Eating Index and Nutrition Information,* Technical Bulletin No. 1866, U.S. Department of Agriculture, Economic Research Service, Washington, D.C., 1998

19 to 50 consumed 4.2 to 4.6 servings of grains per day, while the recommendation is 9 servings.

On average, each gender/age group perceived consuming more fruit servings daily than what was actually the case. Males ages 19 to 50 believed they consumed 2.1 to 2.2 servings of fruit on a given day. Based on their food diaries, they actually consumed less than one serving per day. The recommendation for this group is 4 servings per day.

Adult females believed they consumed more vegetable servings per day than they actually consumed: 2.5 to 2.6 versus 1.7 to 2.2 actual servings. Adult males, on the other hand, believed they consumed slightly less vegetable servings per day than they actually consumed. Both women and men consumed less than the recommendation of 3.5 to 5 servings each day for their gender/age group.

All gender/age groups believed their usual daily milk intake was far more than what they actually consumed. They thought they consumed 2.1 to 3.2 servings or milk products per day, but their food diaries indicated they consumed 1 to 1.6 servings per day.

All gender/age groups perceived their typical servings of meat, poultry, fish, dry beans, eggs, and nuts as more than what they actually consumed. They thought they ate 2.7 to 3.7 servings but their food diaries indicated they consumed only 1.6 to 2.5 servings per day. Meat consumption was also below Pyramid recommendations.

Each gender/age group underestimated its average daily servings of fats, oils, and sweets, perceiving only 1.6

to 2.2 servings versus actually consuming 3.0 to 4.5 servings. The Food Guide Pyramid does not specify the number or size of servings but recommends that people consume these foods sparingly.

The study concluded that people's perceptions of their food group consumption were very different from their actual consumption.

THE HEALTHY EATING INDEX

The Healthy Eating Index (HEI) was developed by the USDA's Center for Nutrition Policy and Promotion (CNPP) to measure and monitor the type and quantity of foods eaten and the extent that nutrition knowledge and diet-health awareness influence diet.

The HEI consists of 10 components, representing different aspects of a healthful diet:

- Components 1–5 measure the degree to which a person's diet conforms to the USDA's Food Guide Pyramid serving recommendations for the five major food groups: grains, vegetables, fruits, milk, and meat.

TABLE 8.5

Diet-health awareness in U.S. households, 1989–90

Question	Yes	No
	Percent	
Have you heard about any health problems that might be related to how much:		
Fat a person eats?	71.3	28.7
Saturated fat a person eats?	58.6	41.4
Fiber a person eats?	48.8	51.2
Salt a person eats?	84.7	15.3
Calcium a person eats?	59.3	40.7
Cholesterol a person eats?	81.7	18.3
Sugar a person eats?	79.6	20.4
Iron a person eats?	47.5	52.5

Note: Based on the 1989–90 Diet Health Knowledge Survey.

SOURCE: Jayachandran Variyam, James Blaylock, David Smallwood, and Peter Basiotis, "Table 4: Diet-health awareness questions and percent responses," in *USDA's Healthy Eating Index and Nutrition Information,* Technical Bulletin No. 1866, U.S. Department of Agriculture, Economic Research Service, Washington, D.C., 1998

FIGURE 8.3

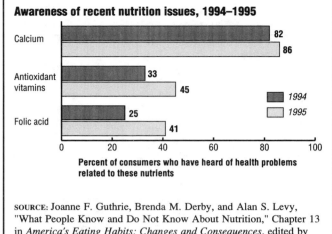

Awareness of recent nutrition issues, 1994–1995

SOURCE: Joanne F. Guthrie, Brenda M. Derby, and Alan S. Levy, "What People Know and Do Not Know About Nutrition," Chapter 13 in *America's Eating Habits: Changes and Consequences,* edited by Elizabeth Frazao, Economic Research Service, U.S. Department of Agriculture, Washington, D.C., 1999

FIGURE 8.4

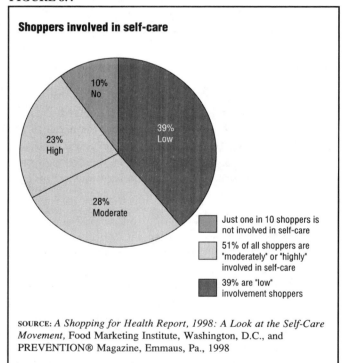

Shoppers involved in self-care

SOURCE: *A Shopping for Health Report, 1998: A Look at the Self-Care Movement,* Food Marketing Institute, Washington, D.C., and PREVENTION® Magazine, Emmaus, Pa., 1998

- Component 6 measures total fat consumption as a percentage of total food energy (calorie) intake.

- Component 7 measures saturated fat consumption as a percentage of total food energy intake.

- Component 8 measures total cholesterol intake.

- Component 9 measures total sodium intake.

- Component 10 measures variety in a person's diet.

The total HEI score is the sum of the 10 components, and the maximum score is 100. An HEI score over 80 indicates a "good" diet; a score between 51 and 80 indicates the diet "needs improvement"; and a score lower than 51 indicates a "poor" diet. The HEI reflects dietary intake in relation to the five major food groups in the Food Guide Pyramid. In developing the Index, the CNPP used the Pyramid's serving recommendations as shown in Table 8.2.

Shanthy Bowman, Mark Lino, Shirley Gerrior, and P. Peter Basiotis, in "The Healthy Eating Index" (*Family Economics and Nutrition Review,* Vol. 11, No. 3, 1998), found that, although the diet quality of Americans had gotten better over the previous 10 years, it still needed much improvement. In fact, in 1996 the diets of most people (70.5 percent) needed improvement. Just 12.2 percent of the population had a good diet, while 17.3 percent had a poor diet. HEI scores from 1996 differed little from those of 1994 and 1995. (See Figure 8.1.)

Julia Dinkins ("Beliefs and Attitudes of Americans Toward Their Diet," *Nutrition Insights,* USDA, June 2000) analyzed dietary data from over 1,800 adults. Nearly one-quarter (23 percent) were interested in improving their diet, compared with 37 percent who were not interested and 40 percent who believed their diet needed no improvement. (See Table 8.3.) Nearly two-thirds (63 percent) of those interested in improving their diet were female. Over one-third (36 percent) of those interested in improving their diet had a household income at or below 130 percent of the poverty threshold, meaning that they were poor or near-poor.

HEI Scores by Population Characteristics

Based on data from the USDA's 1996 *Continuing Survey of Food Intakes by Individuals,* the CNPP looked at Americans' diet quality by race and gender subgroups. The mean HEI score for African Americans was 59, compared with 64

TABLE 8.6

Self-care and shopping habits by segment

	Total Shoppers	High Involvement	Moderate Involvement	Low Involvement	No Involvement
Base Size:	**1,000**	**222**	**287**	**389**	**102**
Compared to 12 months ago:					
More aware of benefits of healthy diet	57%	67%	58%	52%	50%
Eat more healthfully	56%	67%	58%	51%	42%
More likely to treat self	31%	41%	31%	27%	25%
In past month:					
Purchased organic products	21%	37%	19%	16%	9%
Stopped buying product due to ingredient	17%	35%	19%	10%	3%
Started buying product due to ingredient	18%	36%	17%	13%	2%
Things that affect grocery purchases "some" or "a great deal":					
Ensure good health	80%	97%	89%	74%	43%
Reduce fat intake	72%	88%	79%	67%	31%
Reduce/control weight	63%	80%	72%	56%	32%
Reduce cholesterol levels	59%	80%	69%	50%	17%
Follow doctor's advice	55%	76%	69%	43%	20%
Reduce risk of specific health condition	54%	97%	72%	28%	2%
Manage/treat health condition on own	49%	86%	66%	28%	1%
Improve stamina/increase energy	45%	76%	57%	26%	11%
Cope with food intolerances	30%	49%	39%	17%	11%
Manage stress	26%	55%	38%	8%	1%
Enhance athletic performance	26%	48%	27%	16%	7%
Slow down aging process	22%	42%	26%	12%	5%
Manage allergies	22%	46%	28%	9%	—

source: *A Shopping for Health Report, 1998: A Look at the Self-Care Movement,* Food Marketing Institute, Washington, D.C., and *Prevention,* Emmaus, Pa., 1998

TABLE 8.7

Self-care and type of health information sought by segment

	Total Shoppers	High Involvement	Moderate Involvement	Low Involvement	No Involvement
Base Size:	**1,000**	**222**	**287**	**389**	**102**
Information sought in the past month:					
The health benefits of limiting fat intake	27%	43%	30%	21%	9%
The benefits & uses of herbal products	19%	42%	21%	9%	1%
The importance of increasing fiber	19%	32%	22%	13%	2%
Appropriate caloric intake for a person of your age, size & gender	19%	28%	21%	16%	4%
Appropriate uses of natural remedies	19%	40%	22%	8%	1%
The health benefits of reducing salt intake	17%	27%	18%	13%	4%
Benefits of organic products	13%	29%	15%	6%	—
The effects of partially hydrogenated vegetable oils	11%	21%	10%	8%	2%
How to distinguish whole grain products from non-whole grain products	10%	21%	11%	6%	3%
The facts about trans-fatty acids	8%	17%	8%	5%	2%
The health benefits of soy	7%	15%	7%	3%	—

source: *A Shopping for Health Report, 1998: A Look at the Self-Care Movement,* Food Marketing Institute, Washington, D.C., and *Prevention,* Emmaus, Pa., 1998

for whites and 65 for "Other" (comprised of Asian/Pacific Islander Americans, American Indians, and Alaskan Natives). Only 5 percent of African Americans, compared with 11 percent of whites, had a good diet. (See Figure 8.2.)

By age/gender subgroups, children had the highest HEI scores, followed by women 51 years of age or older. HEI scores for teenagers were the lowest across racial groups.

The "Other" racial group often had the highest HEI scores; this may reflect the consumption of more traditional foods and less American convenience or fast foods.

The Effect of Nutrition Knowledge and Diet-Health Awareness

Jayachandran N. Variyam, James Blaylock, David Smallwood, and P. Peter Basiotis, in *USDA's Healthy*

TABLE 8.8

Self-care and factors that motivate purchasing decisions

Percentage of shoppers whose grocery purchases are affected "some" or "a great deal" by the following health concerns

	Total Shoppers	Gender		Age			Education			
		Female	Male	Gen-Xers	Boomers	Matures	< H.S. Grad	H.S. Grad	Some College	College Grad+
Base size	1,000	687	313	238	459	293	96	362	211	327
Motivation										
1. Ensure overall health	80%	83%	74%	76%	82%	81%	61%	77%	87%	86%
2. Reduce fat intake	72%	75%	64%	61%	74%	76%	57%	71%	72%	76%
3. Reduce/control weight	63%	68%	54%	58%	67%	63%	60%	62%	62%	67%
4. Reduce cholesterol levels	59%	62%	51%	43%	63%	65%	52%	56%	58%	64%
5. Following medical advice of doctor	55%	58%	49%	45%	57%	62%	54%	54%	60%	54%
6. Reduce risk of specific health condition	54%	56%	49%	40%	56%	62%	43%	46%	61%	60%
7. Manage/treat own specific health condition	49%	50%	48%	41%	53%	50%	45%	48%	48%	53%
8. Improve stamina/increase energy	45%	45%	43%	42%	47%	43%	34%	38%	49%	51%
9. Cope with food intolerances	30%	31%	27%	25%	32%	31%	21%	30%	30%	32%
10. Manage stress	26%	28%	23%	25%	29%	25%	23%	26%	30%	25%
11. Enhance athletic performance	26%	25%	27%	25%	29%	21%	15%	23%	27%	30%
12. Slow down aging process	22%	24%	18%	14%	24%	25%	21%	20%	22%	24%
13. Manage allergies	22%	24%	16%	19%	24%	20%	22%	19%	21%	25%

SOURCE: *A Shopping for Health Report, 1998: A Look at the Self-Care Movement*, Food Marketing Institute, Washington, D.C., and *Prevention*, Emmaus, Pa., 1998

Eating Index and Nutrition Information (Economic Research Service, USDA, Washington, D.C., 1998), developed a model to measure how nutrition knowledge and diet-health awareness influence an individual's HEI.

Respondents were asked to identify, for example, which of two foods has a higher fiber content: fruit or meat, cornflakes or oatmeal, popcorn or pretzels. They were also asked to identify which foods contain more cholesterol: liver or T-bone steak, butter or margarine, skim or whole milk. Other questions probed knowledge of different kinds of fat, the types of foods that contain cholesterol, and the relationship between fat and cholesterol.

Respondents answered some questions more easily than they did others. Over 90 percent correctly identified whole-wheat bread as containing more fiber than white bread, but only 56 percent knew that kidney beans contained more fiber than lettuce. Likewise, virtually everyone, 95 percent, knew that skim milk has less cholesterol than whole milk, but only 52 percent identified liver as containing more cholesterol than steak. When respondents were asked what kind of fat, saturated or polyunsaturated, is more likely to be a liquid rather than a solid, only 30 percent knew the correct answer. Less than 40 percent of respondents knew that cholesterol is found only in animal products. (See Table 8.4.)

Table 8.5 lists the questions used to measure awareness of diet-health problems. About 85 percent of respondents indicated that they had heard of health problems associated with salt, but less than 50 percent said the same for fiber and iron.

WHAT DO AMERICANS KNOW ABOUT NUTRITION?

Americans are generally aware of diet–disease relationships that have been widely publicized by the media and the government. Joanne Guthrie, Brenda Derby, and Alan Levy, in "What People Know and Do Not Know About Nutrition" (*America's Eating Habits: Changes and Consequences,* USDA, Washington, D.C., 1999), claim that, although Americans are generally knowledgeable about diet–disease relationships, many consumers need help in specific areas, such as dietary fats and cholesterol.

In 1994 and 1995 the Food and Drug Administration's *Health and Diet Survey* asked consumers if they had heard of health problems related to calcium, antioxidant vitamins, and folic acid. In 1995 most (86 percent) respondents were aware of the relationship of calcium to health. Although less than half had heard about health problems related to not eating enough antioxidant vitamins (45 percent) or folic acid (41 percent), these proportions were significantly higher than those in 1994. (See Figure 8.3.)

Consumers, however, often feel frustrated when they receive differing nutrition information. In a USDA survey of meal planners/preparers, more than two in five (over 40 percent) strongly agreed with the statement, "There are so many recommendations about healthy ways to eat, it's hard to know what to believe."

Nutrition Awareness Does Not Necessarily Change Dietary Behavior

Nutrition scientists caution that, just because a person is aware of certain diet–disease relationships, it does not necessarily mean he or she will put this knowledge into

TABLE 8.9

Shoppers' concern about nutritional content, 1996–2000

Question: Would you say you are very concerned, somewhat concerned, not very concerned, or not at all concerned about the nutritional content of what you eat?

	Jan. 2000 Base	Very Concerned					Jan. 2000 Level of Concern		
		Jan. 1996 %	Jan. 1997 %	Jan. 1998 %	Jan. 1999 %	Jan. 2000 %	Very %	Somewhat %	Not Very/ Not At All %
Total	1,000	58	52	50	49	46	46	41	12
Gender									
Men	262	49	41	42	41	40	40	45	14
Women	738	62	56	53	52	49	49	39	12
Work 20+ hrs/wk	391	59	57	51	48	46	46	43	11
Work 0–19 hrs/wk	324	65	54	56	56	52	52	36	12
Type of Household									
With children	367	59	50	52	48	44	44	44	11
Aged 0–6	181	57	51	52	51	44	44	43	13
Aged 7–17	272	60	50	52	49	44	44	44	11
No children	608	58	53	49	49	48	48	39	13
Age									
15–24[1]	94	47	36	40	33	32	32	43	26
25–39	294	54	48	44	48	45	45	48	7
40–49	197	60	55	59	51	50	50	39	11
50–64	236	66	63	54	52	49	49	41	10
65 and older	176	64	47	52	52	49	49	30	19
Region									
East	215	59	54	51	49	47	47	39	13
Midwest	288	55	49	50	45	44	44	40	15
South	299	62	57	55	52	44	44	43	12
West	198	56	43	41	50	52	52	40	8
Education									
High school or less	411	57	47	47	46	40	40	43	17
Some college or more	557	59	55	53	51	52	52	39	9
Medically Restricted Diet									
Yes	209	73	64	65	64	58	58	29	12
No	763	55	49	47	45	43	43	44	13
Vegetarian									
Yes	69	78	74	58	63	57	57	30	13
No	904	57	50	50	47	45	45	41	13

May not add to 100 percent because "not sure" responses are not shown.
Note: Modification to question wording in 2000.
[1]Prior to 2000, youngest age category was 18–24 years.

SOURCE: "Table 40: Shoppers' Concern About Nutritional Content, 1996-2000," in *Trends in the United States: Consumer Attitudes and the Supermarket 2000*, Food Marketing Institute, Washington, D.C., 2000

practice. For example, despite the growing awareness, especially among women, of the relationship between calcium and health, the USDA's 1989–91 and 1994 *Continuing Surveys of Food Intakes by Individuals* found that calcium intake by female respondents ages 20 and over had not improved between these time periods. The women's calcium intake at both time periods remained at 75 percent of the Recommended Dietary Allowances (RDAs).

Other factors may also counteract consumers' nutrition awareness. Many individuals misperceive their actual nutrient intakes. In addition, social and economic factors, such as the rising trend of away-from-home meals, may lead to less consumption of certain nutrients.

SHOPPERS' BEHAVIOR AND SELF-CARE

Each year, the Food Marketing Institute (FMI) and *Prevention* magazine survey food shoppers' attitudes and

behaviors about nutrition, and their effect on food purchases. In 1998 the survey also examined shoppers' interest "in using supermarkets as one-stop centers for health-related products, services, and information" (*A Shopping for Health Report, 1998: A Look at the Self-Care Movement,* Food Marketing Institute and *Prevention* magazine, Washington, D.C., 1998).

Types of Shoppers Based on Involvement in Self-Care

The growing numbers of health information sources have enabled today's consumers to learn more about staying healthy and preventing disease. This means of taking responsibility for one's own health is called "self-care." The FMI and *Prevention* magazine point out that baby boomers (born between 1946 and 1964), who number nearly 80 million adults, or about 40 percent of the adult U.S. population, are the driving force in this self-care movement.

TABLE 8.10

Evaluation of diet, 1996–2000

Question: Thinking of all the foods you eat at home and away from home, how would you describe your diet? Would you say that it could be a lot healthier, could be somewhat healthier, is healthy enough, or is as healthy as it could possibly be?

| | Jan. 2000 Base | Could Be Somewhat or A Lot Healthier | | | | | Jan. 2000 | | | |
		Jan. 1996 %	Jan. 1997 %	Jan. 1998 %	Jan. 1999 %	Jan. 2000 %	A Lot Healthier %	Somewhat Healthier %	Healthy Enough %	Healthy As It Could Possibly Be %
Total	1,000	73	73	70	68	68	22	46	24	8
Gender										
Men	262	74	69	72	69	69	27	42	21	9
Women	738	73	74	68	68	67	20	47	24	8
Work 20+ hrs/wk	391	75	76	74	74	76	20	55	19	5
Work 0–19 hrs/wk	324	71	71	62	62	56	20	36	31	11
Age										
15–24[1]	94	71	75	79	76	69	23	46	26	5
25–39	294	78	80	74	72	77	24	53	19	4
40–49	197	79	77	74	73	73	25	48	22	5
50–64	236	75	65	66	68	69	23	46	21	9
65 and older	176	44	55	51	53	43	14	29	36	19
Income										
$15,000 or less	104	68	72	60	62	61	25	36	18	18
$15,001–$25,000	109	75	73	68	73	78	30	48	16	6
$25,001–$35,000	151	73	71	77	67	69	26	43	22	9
$35,001–$50,000	172	78	77	74	71	73	18	55	19	8
$50,001–$75,000	159	73	77	75	71	71	23	48	26	3
$75,001 or more	125	73	68	63	69	66	18	47	28	6
Type of Household										
With children	367	78	78	76	74	74	23	51	20	5
Aged 0–6	181	76	79	75	72	74	23	51	22	3
Aged 7–17	272	79	77	77	74	75	25	50	19	6
No children	608	69	68	65	65	64	22	42	25	10

May not add to 100 percent because "not sure" responses are not shown.
[1]Prior to 2000, youngest age category was 18–24 years.

SOURCE: "Table 42: Evaluation of Diet, 1996–2000," in *Trends in the United States: Consumer Attitudes & the Supermarket 2000,* Food Marketing Institute, Washington, D.C., 2000

Based on their involvement in self-care, survey respondents were categorized into four groups—shoppers who are "highly involved" in self-care; shoppers who are "moderately involved" in self-care; "low-involvement" shoppers; and "no-involvement" shoppers. Shoppers who are highly involved (23 percent) and those who are moderately involved (28 percent) in self-care made up half the population of food shoppers. Nearly 4 in 10 (39 percent) were low-involvement shoppers, while just 1 in 10 was not involved in self-care. (See Figure 8.4.)

"HIGHLY INVOLVED" SHOPPERS. As indicated above, 23 percent of all shoppers are highly involved in self-care. Shoppers highly involved in self-care were more likely to be between the ages of 40 and 64, to be working women, to live in a dual-income household, to have a college education, and to earn $50,000 or more.

Over two-thirds (67 percent) reported being more aware of the benefits of a healthful diet than they were 12 months ago. Almost all (97 percent) indicated that their desire to reduce the risk of specific health conditions had influenced their grocery purchasing decisions, and nearly

9 in 10 (86 percent) claimed these decisions were also affected by their desire to manage or treat a particular health condition on their own. (See Table 8.6.)

About two-thirds (67 percent) reported eating more healthfully than they did 12 months ago. In fact, nearly 4 in 10 (37 percent) had purchased organic products during the month prior to the survey. (See Table 8.6.)

Highly involved shoppers tended to seek out health information more than other shoppers did. Four in 10 (43 percent, the largest proportions of all shoppers in this segment) had sought information on the health benefits of limiting fat intake and on the benefits and uses of herbal products (42 percent). (See Table 8.7.) They were also more likely to use health services, when offered, at the supermarkets where they shopped most often—about 4 in 5 (79 percent) used healthful recipes and brochures on health and nutrition.

"MODERATELY INVOLVED" SHOPPERS. As indicated in Figure 8.4, 28 percent of shoppers were moderately involved in self-care. The *Shopping for Health* survey found that shoppers who were moderately involved in self-care were the mostly likely to match the profile of the average shopper—female and married. Like all shoppers, typical moderately involved shoppers were 45 years old, with an average household income of $43,400.

Over half (58 percent) of moderately involved shoppers claimed they were more aware of the benefits of a healthful diet than they were 12 months ago. The same percentage reported eating more healthfully than they did 12 months ago. Two-thirds (66 percent) indicated that their grocery purchases were influenced by their desire to manage or treat a particular health condition on their own. (See Table 8.6.)

Besides managing or treating a specific health condition, three in four shoppers moderately involved in self-care reported using supermarket health services, including healthful recipes, nutrition brochures, experts on natural remedies, and health seminars. As with highly involved shoppers, the largest proportion of moderately involved shoppers (30 percent) looked for information during the past month about the health benefits of limiting fat intake. (See Table 8.7.)

"LOW-INVOLVEMENT" SHOPPERS. Low-involvement shoppers made up the largest segment (39 percent) of all shoppers. They tended to live in households with just one adult and/or to have a retired spouse, if married. They were also more likely to have a household income under $35,000 and to be high school graduates or less. Although half (52

TABLE 8.11

Those on whom shoppers rely to ensure that the foods they buy are nutritious

Question: Who do you feel should be primarily responsible for ensuring that the food you buy in your grocery store is nutritious? Please listen to the entire list before answering. Would you say government institutions or agencies, consumer groups/ organizations, manufacturers/food processors, food stores, farmers or yourself as an individual? (Presentation order is rotated. Single response accepted.)
Base: 1,000 Shoppers

	Jan. 1996[1] %	Jan. 1996[2] %	Jan. 1997[1] %	Jan. 1998 %	Jan. 1999 %	Jan. 2000 %
Yourself as an individual	50	42	54	55	28	47
Manufacturers/food processors	29	22	32	26	7	15
Government institutions or agencies	19	14	22	23	5	15
Food stores	13	7	18	16	3	5
Consumer groups/organizations	9	6	14	8	2	5
All/everybody	18	7	6	7	57	8
Farmers	6	1	9	8	1	2
Other (volunteered)	*	1	1	*	1	*
Not sure	*	*	1	1	1	3

* = Less than 0.5 percent.
1996[1] and 1997[1] split sample. Multiple responses accepted.
1996[2] single response accepted.
Note: Through 1998 and in 2000, "all/everybody" was volunteered, therefore 1999 comparison with data may not be valid.
Note: Modification to question wording in 2000.

SOURCE: "Table 47: Those on Whom Shoppers Rely to Ensure That the Foods They Buy are Nutritious," in *Trends in the United States: Consumer Attitudes & the Supermarket 2000*, Food Marketing Institute, Washington, D.C., 2000

FIGURE 8.5

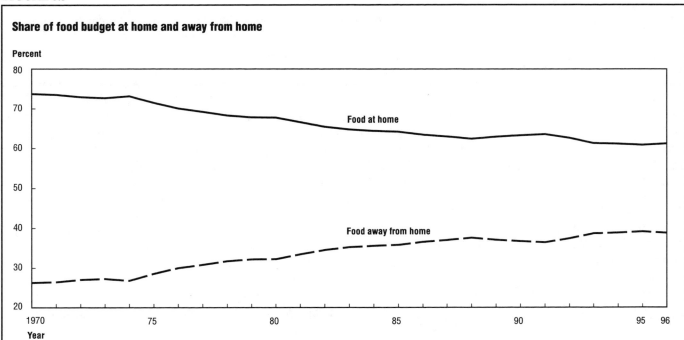

SOURCE: Lin, Biing-Hwan, Fazio, Elizabeth and Guthrie, Joanne, "Figure 1: Share of food budget at home and away from home," in *Away-From-Home Foods Increasingly Important to Quality of American Diet,* Economic Research Service, U.S. Department of Agriculture, Food and Drug Administration, Agricultural Information Bulletin # 749, 2000

TABLE 8.12

Total expenditures on food eaten away from home, 1970–97

Year	Eating and drinking places[1]	Hotels and motels[2]	Retail stores, direct selling[3]	Recreational places[3]	Schools and colleges[4]	All other[5]	Total[6]
			Million dollars				
1970	22,617	1,894	3,325	721	4,475	6,551	39,583
1971	24,166	2,086	3,626	762	4,990	6,621	42,251
1972	27,167	2,390	3,811	832	5,370	7,017	46,587
1973	31,265	2,639	4,218	963	5,605	7,960	52,650
1974	34,029	2,864	4,520	1,167	6,287	9,178	58,045
1975	41,384	3,199	4,952	1,369	7,060	10,145	68,109
1976	47,536	3,769	5,341	1,511	7,854	10,822	76,833
1977	52,491	4,115	5,663	2,606	8,413	11,547	84,835
1978	60,042	4,863	6,323	2,810	9,034	13,012	96,084
1979	68,872	5,551	7,157	2,921	9,914	14,756	109,171
1980	75,883	5,906	8,158	3,040	11,115	16,194	120,296
1981	83,358	6,639	8,830	2,979	11,357	17,751	130,914
1982	90,390	6,888	9,256	2,887	11,692	18,663	139,776
1983	98,710	7,660	9,827	3,271	12,338	19,077	150,883
1984	105,836	8,409	10,315	3,489	12,950	20,047	161,046
1985	111,760	9,168	10,499	3,737	13,534	20,133	168,831
1986	121,699	9,665	11,116	4,059	14,401	20,755	181,695
1987	136,029	11,117	12,121	4,237	14,300	21,122	198,926
1988	149,282	11,905	13,297	4,952	14,929	22,887	217,252
1989	158,604	12,179	14,575	5,841	15,728	24,581	231,508
1990	169,663	12,508	16,223	6,859	16,767	26,189	248,209
1991	173,672	12,460	16,939	7,489	17,959	27,080	255,598
1992	178,939	13,205	17,502	8,401	18,983	27,878	264,908
1993	188,861	13,613	18,334	9,044	20,152	28,456	278,461
1994	195,262	14,416	19,822	9,552	21,434	29,174	289,660
1995	199,349	15,149	21,198	10,402	22,310	29,923	298,331
1996	204,352	16,011	22,897	11,266	23,017	30,680	308,224
1997	211,434	17,447	24,077	11,875	23,756	31,687	320,275

[1]Includes tips.
[2]Includes vending machine operators but not vending machines operated by organizations.
[3]Motion picture theaters, bowling alleys, pool parlors, sport arenas, camps, amusement parks, golf and country clubs (includes concessions beginning in 1977).
[4]Includes school food subsidies.
[5]Military exchanges and clubs; railroad dining cars; airlines; food service in manufacturing plants, institutions, hospitals, boarding houses, fraternities and sororities, and civic and social organizations; and food supplied to military forces, civilian employees, and child daycare.
[6]Computed from unrounded data.

SOURCE: Judith Jones Putnam and Jane E. Allshouse, "Table 104 -- Food eaten away from home: Total expenditures 1970–97" in *Food Consumption, Prices and Expenditures, 1970–1997*, U.S. Department of Agriculture, Washington, D.C., 1998

percent) of low-involvement shoppers reported being more aware of the benefits of a healthful diet than they were 12 months ago, just slightly over one-quarter (28 percent) admitted that a desire to manage a health condition had a bearing on their grocery purchase decisions. (See Table 8.6.)

Unlike shoppers who were highly or moderately involved in self-care, just 2 in 10 (21 percent) low-involvement shoppers sought fat-intake information in the month prior to the survey. (See Table 8.7.) Nonetheless, at least half of the shoppers reported using health services in the supermarkets they frequented. These included requesting health-related products; obtaining healthful recipes and nutrition brochures; and using the services of a nutritionist, an expert on natural remedies, and/or an on-site pharmacist who knew about natural remedies.

"NO-INVOLVEMENT" SHOPPERS. No-involvement shoppers made up just 10 percent of all shoppers. Nearly half

were male, and two in five were between 25 and 39 years old. Compared with shoppers highly involved in self-care, no-involvement shoppers were more likely to live in one-adult households and less likely to have household incomes of $50,000 and higher.

Although just 1 percent of no-involvement shoppers indicated that their grocery purchases were affected by a desire to manage a health condition, nearly one-third (32 percent) reported that fat-intake reduction and weight control were factors that influenced their grocery-buying decisions. (See Table 8.6.) The researchers felt this behavior could be attributed to vanity and not disease prevention.

Generally, no-involvement shoppers showed very little interest in obtaining health information. Nonetheless, half (50 percent) said they were more aware of the benefits of a healthful diet than they were 12 months ago. In addition,

Nutrition: A Key to Good Health

FIGURE 8.6

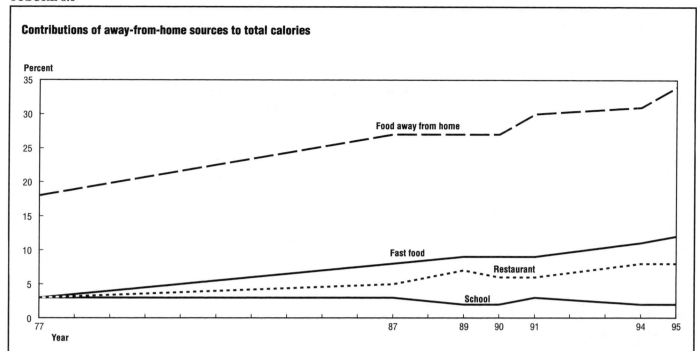

Contributions of away-from-home sources to total calories

SOURCE: Lin, Biing-Hwan, Fazio, Elizabeth and Guthrie, Joanne, "Figure 2: Contributions of away-from-home sources to total calories," in *Away-From-Home Foods Increasingly Important to Quality of American Diet,* Economic Research Service, U.S. Department of Agriculture, Food and Drug Administration, Agricultural Information Bulletin # 749, 2000

about 4 in 10 (42 percent) reported they were eating more healthfully than 12 months ago. (See Table 8.6.)

Shoppers Seek Health-Related Information

As Americans take on more responsibility for their health, they are seeking more information on diet, nutrition, and health. The *Shopping for Health* survey found that, among shoppers looking for health-related information, the largest proportion (27 percent) wanted information on the health benefits of limiting fat intake. About one-fifth (19 percent) each sought information on the benefits and uses of herbal products, the importance of increasing fiber intake, appropriate caloric intake, and the appropriate uses of natural remedies.

Self-Care Influences Grocery Purchases

As shoppers become more knowledgeable about diet, nutrition, and health, they are more likely to put this information into practice. According to the researchers in *A Shopping for Health Report, 1998: A Look at the Self-Care Movement* (Food Marketing Institute and *Prevention* magazine, Washington, D.C., 1998), "Shoppers aren't just saying they are health-oriented. In nearly every case, those who report their grocery purchases are affected by the health concerns measured in the study are also significantly more likely to be eating more healthfully than they were 12 months earlier." About half of the respondents reported that a desire to reduce the risk of a specific health condition (54 percent of respondents) or to manage/treat a specific health condition on their own (49 percent) were factors that influenced their purchasing decisions. (See Table 8.8.)

About 7 in 10 (72 percent) shoppers reported that their purchasing decisions were at least somewhat affected by the desire to reduce fat intake. About 6 in 10 were motivated by the desire to reduce/control weight (63 percent) or reduce their cholesterol levels (59 percent). Women were more likely than men, and generation-Xers (ages 18 to 33) were less likely than baby boomers (ages 34 to 52) and "matures" (age 53 and over), to say these three factors affected what they bought at the supermarket. (See Table 8.8.)

CONSUMERS' CONCERN WITH NUTRITION

In the Food Marketing Institute's annual survey of shopping behavior, 1,000 shoppers are asked about their concern with the nutritional content of what they eat. Among both genders, and in all age groups, types of households and regions, there was a decrease in the number of people "very concerned" about nutritional content from 1996 to 2000. (See Table 8.9.)

When asked about the food they eat at home and away from home, 68 percent of respondents said that their diets could be "somewhat" or "a lot" healthier. Again, in most categories, this represented a decrease from 1996.

TABLE 8.13

Fat and saturated fat intake levels and nutrient densities of foods at home and away from home, 1977–1995

Nutrient	1977-78	1987-88	1989	1990	1991	1994	1995
Fat				*Grams*			
Average daily intake	86.3	74.7	72.0	72.9	73.4	74.9	76.2
				Percent of calories			
Average intake	41.1	37.0	35.3	35.4	35.1	33.6	33.6
				Percent			
People meeting recommendation[1]	13	21	30	29	30	36	37
				Percent of calories			
Benchmark density[1]	30.0	30.0	30.0	30.0	30.0	30.0	30.0
Average fat density	41.2	37.0	35.3	35.4	35.1	33.6	33.6
Home foods	41.1	36.3	34.4	34.5	33.8	31.9	31.5
Away-from-home foods[2]	41.2	38.7	37.8	38.1	38.2	37.4	37.6
Restaurants	46.2	41.3	40.7	40.7	41.2	40.0	40.1
Fast-food places	41.6	39.7	39.7	39.6	38.8	39.9	39.3
Schools[3]	40.1	38.0	37.7	36.1	36.8	36.1	35.7
Other public places	41.4	41.2	34.8	40.9	42.3	30.3	32.6
Others	38.6	36.4	33.9	33.1	34.2	34.1	34.9
Saturated fat				*Grams*			
Average daily intake	na	27.7	25.7	26.0	26.0	25.6	26.2
				Percent of calories			
Average intake	na	13.8	12.6	12.6	12.4	11.5	11.5
				Percent			
People meeting recommendation[1]	na	17	29	29	31	40	39
Nutrient density				*Percent of calories*			
Benchmark density[1]	na	10.0	10.0	10.0	10.0	10.0	10.0
Average sat. fat density	na	13.8	12.6	12.6	12.4	11.5	11.5
Home foods	na	13.5	12.3	12.2	12.1	11.1	10.9
Away-from-home foods[2]	na	14.7	13.5	13.8	13.3	12.4	12.8
Restaurants	na	15.5	14.3	13.5	14.0	12.3	12.5
Fast-food places	na	15.4	14.2	14.5	13.1	13.6	13.8
Schools[3]	na	13.9	15.4	16.1	15.4	14.4	14.2
Other public places	na	15.2	12.0	14.6	13.8	9.8	9.8
Others	na	13.7	12.0	11.8	12.0	11.1	12.1

na = not available.

[1] Recommendations are 30 percent or less of calories from fat and less than 10 percent of calories from saturated fat. These recommendations are the benchmark densities.

[2] Away from home presents the aggregate of fast foods, restaurants, schools, other public places, and others.

[3] Schools are classified as a separate category for children only; adults are included in "others."

SOURCE: Lin, Biing-Hwan, Fazio, Elizabeth and Guthrie, Joanne, "Table 6: Fat and saturated fat intake levels and nutrient densities of foods at home and away from home, 1977-95," in *Away-From-Home Foods Increasingly Important to Quality of American Diet,* Economic Research Service, U.S. Department of Agriculture, Food and Drug Administration, Agricultural Information Bulletin # 749, 2000

Almost a quarter (24 percent) responded that their diets were "healthy enough." (See Table 8.10.)

In 2000 close to half (47 percent) of respondents felt that they, themselves, should be primarily responsible for ensuring that the food they buy is nutritious. Only 15 percent felt that this was the responsibility of food manufacturers and processors, down from 29 percent in 1996. (See Table 8.11.)

EATING OUT

The changing American scene—more women in the workforce, the increasing number of dual-earner households, smaller families (many consisting of empty-nester baby boomers)—is reflected in America's eating habits. Americans are eating out more often. In 1997 *Tableservice Restaurant Trends* (National Restaurant Association, Washington, D.C., 1997) reported that, for nearly 4 in 10 adults, restaurant meals were essential to the way they lived.

The National Restaurant Association, a trade association of more than 30,000 members representing over 175,000 restaurants, is the leading source for research and information on the restaurant industry. In 1996 a nationwide survey by the association (*Meal Consumption Behavior,* Washington, D.C., 1996) found that the typical American (eight years old or older) ate an average of 4.1 commercially prepared (away-from-home) meals per week, up from 3.7 meals in 1981. Meanwhile, privately prepared (at-home) meals decreased from an average of 15.1 meals per week in 1981 to 14.4 in 1996.

USDA data on the share of food budgets confirms this. In 1970, 26 percent of total food expenditures were away from home; by 1996 that number had risen to 39 percent. (See Figure 8.5.) The percent of the American food budget spent on food at home has been declining since 1970, while the share spent on food away from home has been increasing. Total expenditures on food away from home have risen from $39.6 million in 1970 to

FIGURE 8.7

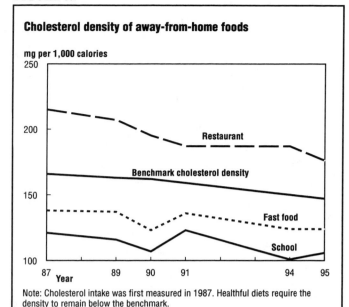

Cholesterol density of away-from-home foods

mg per 1,000 calories

Restaurant

Benchmark cholesterol density

Fast food

School

Note: Cholesterol intake was first measured in 1987. Healthful diets require the density to remain below the benchmark.

SOURCE: Lin, Biing-Hwan, Fazio, Elizabeth and Guthrie, Joanne, "Figure 8: Cholesterol density of away-from-home foods," in *Away-From-Home Foods Increasingly Important to Quality of American Diet,* Economic Research Service, U.S. Department of Agriculture, Food and Drug Administration, Agricultural Information Bulletin # 749, 2000

FIGURE 8.8

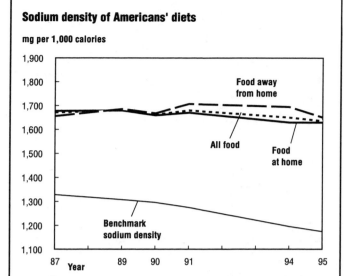

Sodium density of Americans' diets

mg per 1,000 calories

Food away from home

All food

Food at home

Benchmark sodium density

Note: Sodium intake was first measured in 1987. Healthful diets require the density to remain below the benchmark.

SOURCE: Lin, Biing-Hwan, Fazio, Elizabeth and Guthrie, Joanne, "Figure 9: Sodium density of Americans' diets," in *Away-From-Home Foods Increasingly Important to Quality of American Diet,* Economic Research Service, U.S. Department of Agriculture, Food and Drug Administration, Agricultural Information Bulletin # 749, 2000

FIGURE 8.9

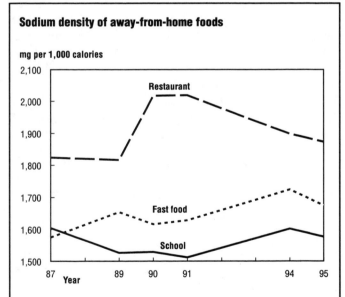

Sodium density of away-from-home foods

mg per 1,000 calories

Restaurant

Fast food

School

Note: Sodium was first measured in 1987. Healthful diets require the density to remain below the benchmark; the benchmark was 1,175 mg per 1,000 calories in 1995.

SOURCE: Lin, Biing-Hwan, Fazio, Elizabeth and Guthrie, Joanne, "Figure 10: Sodium density of away-from-home foods," in *Away-From-Home Foods Increasingly Important to Quality of American Diet,* Economic Research Service, U.S. Department of Agriculture, Food and Drug Administration, Agricultural Information Bulletin # 749, 2000

FIGURE 8.10

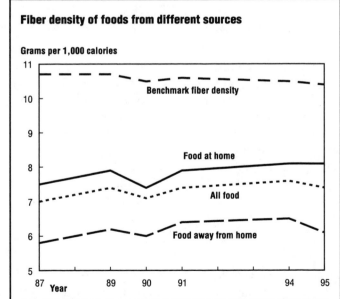

Fiber density of foods from different sources

Grams per 1,000 calories

Benchmark fiber density

Food at home

All food

Food away from home

Note: Dietary fiber was first measured in 1987. Healthful diets require the density to be above the benchmark.

SOURCE: Lin, Biing-Hwan, Fazio, Elizabeth and Guthrie, Joanne, "Figure 13: Fiber density of foods from different sources," in *Away-From-Home Foods Increasingly Important to Quality of American Diet,* Economic Research Service, U.S. Department of Agriculture, Food and Drug Administration, Agricultural Information Bulletin # 749, 2000

FIGURE 8.11

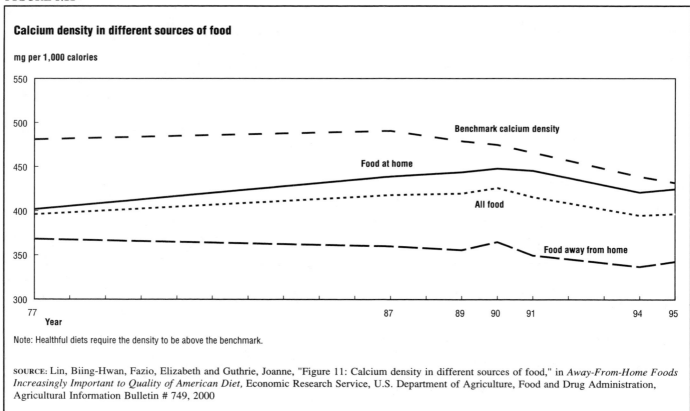

Calcium density in different sources of food

mg per 1,000 calories

Benchmark calcium density

Food at home

All food

Food away from home

Year: 77 · · · 87 · 89 · 90 · 91 · · · 94 · 95

Note: Healthful diets require the density to be above the benchmark.

SOURCE: Lin, Biing-Hwan, Fazio, Elizabeth and Guthrie, Joanne, "Figure 11: Calcium density in different sources of food," in *Away-From-Home Foods Increasingly Important to Quality of American Diet,* Economic Research Service, U.S. Department of Agriculture, Food and Drug Administration, Agricultural Information Bulletin # 749, 2000

$320.3 million in 1997—an astonishing 709 percent increase. (See Table 8.12.)

Eating-Out Trend May Lower Nutritional Quality of American Diets

TOTAL CALORIES. Biing-Hwan Lin, Joanne Guthrie, and Elizabeth Frazão, in "Away From Home Food Increasingly Important to Quality of American Diet" (*USDA Agricultural Information Bulletin 749,* Washington, D.C., 2000), reported that, over the past two decades, the proportion of total calories consumed in away-from-home meals increased. In 1977–78, food away from home (food consumed in fast-food places, restaurants, schools, and other public places) accounted for 18 percent of the total caloric intake. By 1995 eating out contributed to 34 percent of total caloric intake.

In addition, the share of calories eaten at fast-food places (3 percent) and restaurants (3 percent) in 1977–78 rose to 12 percent and 8 percent, respectively, in 1995. (See Figure 8.6.) According to the USDA, consumers may not be as careful in monitoring their caloric consumption when eating out—they tend to consume more food or to eat higher-calorie food.

TOTAL FAT, SATURATED FAT, AND CHOLESTEROL. The *Dietary Guidelines for Americans* recommends that total fat intake be limited to no more than 30 percent of total

calories and to no more than 10 percent of calories from saturated fats. These percentages are the "benchmark densities" for the two substances. Since 1977 Americans have decreased the total fat density of food consumed both at home and away from home. However, while the total fat density for food eaten at home declined significantly between 1977–78 and 1995, from 41.1 percent to 31.5 percent, fat density for away-from-home food declined just slightly during the same period, from 41.2 percent to 37.6 percent. (See Table 8.13.)

While all foods have dropped in fat content, only foods eaten at home in 1995 approached the 30-percent benchmark for dietary calories from fat. Foods eaten away from home remained at 32 to 40 percent fat content. (See Table 8.13.)

The National Research Council recommends a daily cholesterol intake of no more than 300 milligrams (mg) or about 166 mg per 1,000 calories, regardless of age, gender, or total caloric intake. As with saturated fat, the cholesterol content of Americans' diets was first measured in 1987–88. Since then, average cholesterol density has been lower than the 300-mg benchmark density, but restaurant food exceeds that density. (Figure 8.7.)

SODIUM. The National Research Council recommends that daily sodium intake not exceed 2,400 mg, regardless of age or gender. Nonetheless, American sodium intakes remain above recommended levels. (See Figure 8.8.) While away-from-home foods generally contain more sodium than at-home foods, restaurant foods contain much more sodium than any other type of away-from-home food and are much higher than the benchmark sodium density of 1,175 mg per 1,000 calories. (See Figure 8.9.)

DIETARY FIBER. Although fiber densities for home and away-from-home foods have increased slightly since 1987, they have stayed far below the benchmark density of 10.5 grams per 1,000 calories. In 1995 foods consumed at home had a fiber density of 8.1 grams per 1,000 calories; those eaten away from home had a fiber density of 6.1 grams per 1,000 calories. (See Figure 8.10.) Health authorities are concerned that the rising frequency of eating out may offset the little progress made in increased fiber intake at home.

CALCIUM AND IRON. In 1995 away-from-home food had a calcium density of 343 mg per 1,000 calories—well below the benchmark density of 425 mg per 1,000 calories. (See Figure 8.11.)

Between 1977 and 1995, the iron density of at-home foods increased more rapidly than that of food consumed away from home. In 1995, three in five (61 percent) of all individuals satisfied their recommended iron intake, compared with two in five persons (42 percent) in 1977–78. The USDA attributes this trend partly to the increased home consumption of iron-fortified breakfast cereals.

On the other hand, the increasing practice of eating out might have contributed to lower iron intake among some women—in 1995 only one in every three women ages 18 to 39 met her recommended iron intake. For these women, foods eaten away from home accounted for 6 mg of dietary iron per 1,000 calories, compared with 8.2 mg for at-home foods. The benchmark density was 8.4 mg per 1,000 calories.

The Perception and Reality of Eating Out

The USDA points out that consumers seem to pay more attention to the nutritional properties of at-home foods than away-from-home foods. Although many people claim that nutritious foods are important to them, their eating-out practices do not support this claim.

The National Restaurant Association conducted a nationwide survey to find out if "concerns about health and nutrition influence the choice of restaurants and foods eaten away from home" (*Nutrition and Restaurants: A Consumer Perspective,* Washington, D.C., 1993). The survey asked how likely it was that the respondent would order specific foods. Most respondents (86 percent) indicated they would likely try fresh fruit at a restaurant if it were available. At least 80 percent claimed they would likely eat skinless poultry, Italian dishes, fruit salad, and broiled or baked fish or seafood. Also included in the top-ten food items most likely to be ordered were main-dish salads with vegetables and grains, Chinese dishes, steak or roast beef, and whole-grain muffins. The foods that the respondents thought they would be least likely to try included raw fish or shellfish, caffeine-free coffee, Greek dishes, and sugar substitutes.

The foods that consumers actually did order during 1993 revealed some major discrepancies between what they said they would try and what they ordered. The most commonly ordered foods were hamburgers (87 percent) and steak or roast beef (84 percent). Fresh fruit (83 percent) was the number three item ordered, followed by broiled or baked fish or seafood, French fries, and Italian dishes, all at 78 percent. The National Restaurant Association concluded that "consumers generally overstated their likelihood of trying foods lower in fat and calories while understating their likelihood of ordering foods that are high in fat and calories."

REASONS FOR THE DISCREPANCY. The USDA offers two reasons for the discrepancy between consumer perception and reality when it comes to eating out:

• Consumers may have different attitudes about food consumed away from home than food eaten at home. They may think that it is not as important to consider the nutritional quality of away-from-home food, or they might be less willing to give up taste when eating out. Although Americans are eating out far more often than they used to, they may still feel that eating out represents a treat, an occasion when they don't have to concern themselves with nutrition. Americans may not realize that away-from-home foods have become an integral part of their diets.

• Traditional nutrition education has been geared toward the purchase and preparation of home foods—for example, the advice to cook without added fat. When it comes to foods eaten outside the home, nutritional properties may not be as apparent to consumers. For one thing, consumers may not prepare at home the foods they order when eating out. Additionally, consumers can't see the amount of fat used by restaurant cooks. Finally, restaurants often serve much larger portions of food than Americans would serve and consume at home.

CHAPTER 9

WEIGHT, DIET, AND EXERCISE

Americans are obsessed with weight. Tall, slender models (male and female), seen in every form of visual advertising, make many people feel inadequate. Nonetheless, the Centers for Disease Control and Prevention (CDC) report an upward trend in the prevalence of overweight and obesity among the American people. According to the *Third National Health and Nutrition Examination Survey* (NHANES III), the prevalence of obesity in adults increased from nearly 13 percent in 1960 to 22.5 percent of the U.S. population in 1994, with most of the increase occurring during the 1990s.

PREVALENCE OF OVERWEIGHT

The National Center for Health Statistics (NCHS) of the CDC periodically surveys Americans to provide data and prevalence estimates for a variety of health measures. The NHANES program has collected weight data in three surveys (1976 to 1980, 1988 to 1991, and 1991 to 1994). Beginning in 1999 NHANES became a continuous annual survey. The survey used the body mass index (BMI) as a measure of weight relative to a person's height. The NHANES defined overweight as a BMI of 27.8 or higher for men and a BMI of 27.3 or higher for women.

NHANES III found that substantial proportions of adults were overweight in the United States—33.3 percent of men and 36.4 percent of women. While the proportions of overweight men from different racial and ethnic groups were about the same, half or more black and Mexican American women were overweight, compared to one-third of white women. (See Table 9.1.)

The Bureau of the Census, using NHANES III and NHANES 1999 data, found that 35 percent of U.S. adults were overweight and 26 percent were obese. (See Table 9.2.) In 1996 nearly half (44.2 percent) of males between 50 and 69 were overweight, compared to 39.8 percent of women of the same age group.

TABLE 9.1

Number and percentage of adults over age 20 who were overweight[1], by sex and race/ethnicity[2]—as reported in Third National Health and Nutrition Examination Survey (NHANES III), 1988-1994

	No.	(%)	(95% CI[3])
Men			
White, non-Hispanic	3,285	(33.7)	(31.9%–35.4%)
Black, non-Hispanic	2,112	(33.3)	(31.2%–35.1%)
Mexican American	2,250	(36.4)	(33.2%–39.1%)
Total	**7,933**	**(33.3)**	**(31.5%–34.8%)**
Women[4]			
White, non-Hispanic	3,755	(33.5)	(31.3%–35.5%)
Black, non-Hispanic	2,490	(52.3)	(48.9%–55.2%)
Mexican American	2,128	(50.1)	(47.6%–52.3%)
Total	**8,748**	**(36.4)**	**(34.5%–38.0%)**
Total[5]	**16,681**	**(34.9)**	**(33.6%–36.1%)**

[1] Overweight is defined as body mass index (kg/m^2) $\geq$ 27.8 for men and $\geq$ 27.3 for women (85th percentiles from NHANES II for ages 20–29 years). The prevalence of overweight among persons aged 18–19 years, using these criteria, is 15.3% for males and 19.2% for females.
[2] Numbers for other racial/ethnic groups were too small for meaningful analysis.
[3] Confidence interval.
[4] Excludes pregnant women.
[5] Total estimates include racial/ethnic groups not shown.

SOURCE: "Table 9.1: Number and percentage of adults (aged > 20 years) who were overweight, by sex and race/ethnicity--United States, Third National Health and Nutrition Examination Survey (NHANES III), 1988-94," in "Update: Prevalence of Overweight Among Children, Adolescents, and Adults--United States, 1988-94," in *Morbidity and Mortality Weekly Report*, Centers for Disease Control and Prevention, Atlanta, GA, Vol. 46, No. 9, March 7, 1997

Overweight Children

A child is considered obese when his or her weight exceeds his or her ideal weight, which is based on age, height, and body frame, by 20 percent. In 1998 U.S. Surgeon General David Satcher declared childhood obesity an epidemic in the United States. At least one in five American children are overweight, and the number of overweight children continues to grow. NHANES IV

TABLE 9.2

Age-adjusted* prevalence of overweight and obesity among U.S. adults, by percentage of population, age 20 years and over

	NHANES III (1988-94) (n=16,679)	NHANES 1999 (n=1,615)
Overweight or obese (BMI greater than or equal to 25.0)	56	61
Overweight (BMI 25.0-29.9)	33	35
Obese (BMI greater than or equal to 30.0)	23	26

*Age-adjusted by the direct method to the year 2000 U.S. Bureau of the Census estimates using the age groups 20-29, 30-39, 40-49, 50-59, 60-69, 70-79, and 80 years and over.
Note: NHANES=National Health and Nutrition Examination Survey. BMI=body mass index.

SOURCE: "Table 1: Age-adjusted* prevalance of overweight and obesity among U.S. adults, age 20 years and over," in *Prevalance of Overweight and Obesity Among Adults: United States, 1999,* Centers for Disease Control and Prevention, National Center for Health Statistics, Hyattsville, Md.

TABLE 9.3

Prevalence of overweight among children and adolescents ages 6–19 years, by percentage, for selected years 1963–1965 through 1999

Age (years)[1]	1963-65 1966-70[2]	1971-74	1976-80	1988-94	1999
6-11	4	4	7	11	13
12-19	5	6	5	11	14

[1]Excludes pregnant women starting with 1971-74. Pregnancy status not available for 1963-65 and 1966-70.
[2]Data for 1963-65 are for children 6-11 years of age; data for 1966-70 are for adolescents 12-17 years of age, not 12-19 years.

SOURCE: "Table 1: Prevalence of overweight among children and adolescents ages 6-19 years, for selected years 1963-65 through 1999," in *Prevalence of Overweight Among Children and Adolescents: United States, 1999,* Centers for Disease Control and Prevention, National Center for Health Studies, Hyattsville, Md., 1999

TABLE 9.4

Determing body mass index from height and weight

Body Mass Index (kg/m²)														
Height (in.) 19	20	21	22	23	24	25	26	27	28	29	30	35	40
Body Weight (lb.)													
58	91	96	100	105	110	115	119	124	129	134	138	143	167	191
59	94	99	104	109	114	119	124	128	133	138	143	148	173	198
60	97	102	107	112	118	123	128	133	138	143	148	153	179	204
61	100	106	111	116	122	127	132	137	143	148	153	158	185	211
62	104	109	115	120	126	131	136	124	147	153	158	164	191	218
63	107	113	118	124	130	135	141	146	152	158	163	169	197	225
64	110	116	122	128	134	140	145	151	157	163	169	174	204	232
65	114	120	126	132	138	144	150	156	162	168	171	180	210	240
66	118	124	130	136	142	148	155	161	167	173	179	186	215	247
67	121	127	134	140	146	153	159	166	172	178	185	191	223	255
68	125	131	138	144	151	158	164	171	177	184	190	197	230	262
69	128	135	142	149	155	162	169	176	182	189	196	203	236	270
70	132	139	146	153	160	167	174	181	188	195	202	207	243	278
71	136	143	150	157	165	172	179	186	193	200	208	215	250	286
72	140	147	154	162	169	177	184	191	199	206	213	221	258	294
73	144	151	159	166	174	182	189	197	204	212	219	227	265	302
74	148	155	163	171	179	186	194	202	210	218	225	233	272	311
75	152	160	168	176	184	192	200	208	216	224	232	240	279	319
76	156	164	172	180	189	197	205	213	221	230	238	246	287	328

SOURCE: "Determining Body Mass Index From Height and Weight," in *Clinical Guidelines on the Identification, Evaluation, and Treatment of Overweight and Obesity in Adults, 1998,* National Institutes of Health, National Heart, Lung and Blood Institute

(begun in 1999) found that approximately 13 percent of younger children and 14 percent of adolescents were overweight. Note how the prevalence of overweight children and adolescents has grown since the 1963–1965 survey. (See Table 9.3.)

According to the National Institute of Diabetes and Digestive and Kidney Diseases (NIDDK), the part of the National Institutes of Health (NIH) chiefly responsible for obesity research, children become overweight for several reasons. Children whose parents or siblings are over-

weight are more likely to be overweight. Although heredity plays a role in overweight and obesity, shared family behaviors, such as eating habits and activity levels, also influence a child's weight.

Overweight children tend to eat foods high in fats and calories. An inactive lifestyle further contributes to overweight because children do not burn off the excess calories. The average American child spends about 24 hours each week watching television. In addition, sitting in front of computers and playing video games has taken more time away from physical activities.

Childhood Obesity and Type Two Diabetes

Type Two diabetes, also known as adult-onset diabetes, generally occurs in people over 40. Today, this disease is increasingly diagnosed in obese children, some younger than 10 years old. Type Two diabetes is incurable and degenerative, causing kidney disease, blindness, frequent infection, and cardiovascular complications.

OVERWEIGHT AND OBESITY

In May 1998 the National Heart, Lung, and Blood Institute (NHLBI; also a part of NIH) and the NIDDK released the first federal guidelines on the identification, evaluation, and treatment of overweight and obesity. The NHLBI and NIDDK reported that 97 million overweight Americans—55 percent of the population—are at increased risk for serious medical conditions, including higher rates of certain types of cancer.

The federal standards for being overweight or obese are based on a tool called the body mass index, or BMI. The BMI uses a mathematical formula, incorporating a person's body weight and height to establish a value that determines his or her health risks. Scientists calculate the BMI by dividing a person's weight in kilograms by height in meters squared (kg/m^2. Table 9.4 has done the mathematical calculation and metric conversions to pounds and inches. Table 9.5 shows how to calculate BMI.

The new federal guidelines define overweight as a BMI of 25 to 29.9 and obesity as a BMI of 30 and above. This redefinition of overweight is based on research that relates BMI to risk of death and illness, and supports the *Dietary Guidelines for Americans*. The revised definition is consistent with the definition used by other countries and the World Health Organization (WHO).

BMI numbers apply to both men and women. The new definition also means that many more Americans—about 29 million—previously considered at normal weight are now reclassified as overweight. In June 1998, a month after the new guidelines for overweight were released, the American Heart Association announced that obesity is now considered a major risk factor for a heart attack, not just a contributing risk as previously described.

A person's waist circumference is associated with abdominal fat. A waist circumference of over 40 inches in men and over 35 inches in women, along with a BMI of 25 to 34.9, means an increased risk of disease. The disease risks increase for obese and extremely obese individuals. (See Table 9.6.)

CAUSES OF OBESITY

The panel of NHLBI and NIDDK experts that developed the first federal obesity guidelines defines obesity as "a complex multifactorial chronic disease that develops

TABLE 9.5

How to calculate Body Mass Index (BMI)

$$BMI = \frac{weight\ (in\ kilograms)}{height\ (in\ meters)^2}$$

$$BMI = \frac{weight\ (in\ pounds)\ x\ 705}{height\ (in\ inches)^2}$$

SOURCE: "Figure 9.1: How to Calculate BMI," Center for Nutrition Policy and Promotion, U.S. Department of Agriculture, Washington D.C.

from an interaction of genotype and the environment." The National Institutes of Health believe that "increasing physiologic, biochemical and genetic evidence suggests that overweight is not a simple problem of will power as is sometimes implied, but is a complex disorder of appetite regulation and energy metabolism."

Genetics

In 1994 scientists discovered a genetic mutation that may contribute to overweight. The mutation, first found in obese mice and then in humans, is thought to be responsible for at least some types of obesity. When mice with the defective gene, called "ob" for obese, were injected with leptin, a hormone normally secreted by fat cells, they underwent spectacular weight loss. Leptin caused even normal-weight mice to become thin. Initially, researchers hoped that the process would be the same in humans and that leptin was the missing key to weight control. Further research, however, found that, unlike the "ob" mice who had no detectable levels of leptin, obese humans had leptin levels 20 to 30 times greater than did normal-weight humans.

Scientists have speculated that the normal sequence of events is as follows: Fat cells produce leptin, which travels through the bloodstream to leptin receptors located in the hypothalamus, the portion of the brain that regulates unconscious body functions. If high levels of leptin are received, the receptor passes on a message of too much fat. The brain responds by reducing the appetite or increasing the rate at which fat is burned, or both.

Experts hypothesize that the problem in obese people may lie with leptin receptors that fail to send messages to the brain to stop eating. In addition, chronic high-fat diets may cause leptin insensitivity, creating a vicious cycle where the more the person eats, the less he or she is able to detect when the body is satisfied.

The NIDDK notes there is growing evidence that obesity may have a genetic cause. The NIDDK cites a study of adults who were adopted as children. The study found that the subjects' adult weights were closer to the weights of their biological parents than to their adoptive parents' weights. However, the role of genetics in overweight and

TABLE 9.6

Classification of overweight and obesity by Body Mass Index (BMI), waist circumference, and associated disease risk

	BMI (kg/m²)	Obesity Class	Disease Risk* Relative to Normal Weight & Waist Circumference	
			Men: ≤ 102 cm (≤ 40 in) Women: ≤ 88 cm (≤ 35 in)	Men: > 102 cm (> 40 in) Women: > 88 cm (> 35 in)
Underweight	<18.5			
Normal	18.5-24.9			
Overweight	25.0-29.9		Increased	High
Obesity	30.0-34.9	I	High	Very High
	35.0-39.9	II	Very High	Very High
Extreme Obesity	≥40	III	Extremely High	Extremely High

*Disease risk for type 2 diabetes, hypertension and cardiovascular disease.

SOURCE: "Classification of Overweight and Obesity by BMI, Waist Circumference, and Associated Disease Risk," in *Clinical Guidelines on the Identification, Evaluation, and Treatment of Overweight and Obesity in Adults, 1998,* National Institutes of Health, National Heart, Lung and Blood Institute

obesity remains controversial, and more research is needed to study the link between heredity and weight loss, gain, and maintenance.

Environmental Factors

Researchers warn that no one knows what proportion of a population's obesity is actually caused by heredity. Leah Garnett, in "Is Obesity All in the Genes?" (*Harvard Health Letter,* Vol. 21, No. 6, April 1996), observed, "Environmental factors are the weightiest determinants of who gets fat and who doesn't." The rate of obesity keeps rising, and yet the human gene pool has remained largely unchanged for several generations. Garnett believes that people with a genetic propensity for obesity live in an environment where excess is the norm. Because of this, they will probably gain more weight than people with a tendency toward leanness.

Many experts attribute the increasing proportions of overweight people to the environment they live in. This includes lifestyle behaviors, such as eating habits and physical activity levels. Americans are eating out more. Restaurants not only serve bigger portions to attract patrons, but also tend to serve foods higher in fat.

Modern technology has also affected our weight gain. Computers and televisions encourage a sedentary lifestyle. Even the remote control prevents the expenditure of energy, however minimal, of getting up to adjust a television or stereo dial. Social occasions typically revolve around eating, and sports events do not just involve the perennial hot dogs, but also high-calorie tailgate meals.

Psychological Factors

Psychological factors may also affect eating habits. Some people reach for food in response to stress. Others react to negative emotions, such as boredom, anger, or sadness, by overeating. Studies show that about 30 percent of people who are being treated for serious weight

TABLE 9.7

Overweight and obesity risk factors

Overweight and obesity are known risk factors for:

- diabetes,
- heart disease,
- stroke,
- hypertension,
- gallbladder disease,
- osteoarthritis (degeneration of cartilage and bone of joints),
- sleep apnea and other breathing problems, and
- some forms of cancer (uterine, breast, colorectal, kidney, and gallbladder).

Obesity is associated with:

- high blood cholesterol,
- complications of pregnancy,
- menstrual irregularities,
- hirsutism (presence of excess body and facial hair),
- stress incontinence (urine leakage caused by weak pelvic-floor muscles),
- psychological disorders such as depression, and
- increased surgical risk.

SOURCE: *Statistics Related to Overweight and Obesity,* National Institutes of Health, Weight Control Information Network, Publication 96-4158, 2000

problems are binge eaters. During binge eating episodes, individuals consume large quantities of food, at the same time feeling they cannot control how much they are eating. Those who have severe binge eating problems are said to have a binge eating disorder.

Other Causes

Certain drugs, such as steroids and antidepressants, may cause weight gain. Some illnesses, including depression, and hormonal disorders such as hypothyroidism (loss of activity in the thyroid gland, often characterized by lower metabolism) and Cushing's syndrome (symptoms caused by overactivity of the adrenal glands' outer layers, or cortices) can predispose a person to overeat. About 1 percent of overweight cases results from these causes.

FIGURE 9.1

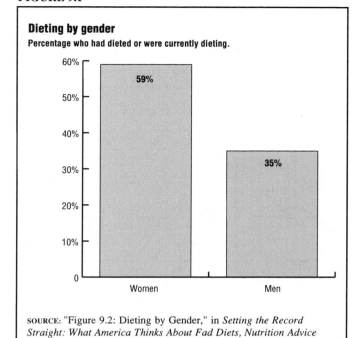

FIGURE 9.2

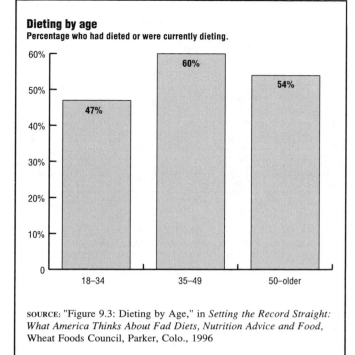

CONSEQUENCES OF OBESITY

Health Risks

New analysis of the NHANES III found that as BMI levels rise, blood pressure and total cholesterol levels increase, and HDL or "good" cholesterol levels decrease. Men in the highest obesity category have more than twice the risk of hypertension (high blood pressure), high blood cholesterol, or both, compared to men with normal weight. Women in the highest obesity category have four times the risk of either or both of these health-risk factors. High blood pressure is a major risk factor for heart disease and stroke. Very high levels of cholesterol and triglycerides (blood fats) can also lead to heart disease.

Other diseases and health problems associated with obesity include hypertension; Type Two diabetes; gallbladder disease; osteoarthritis (deterioration of the joints); respiratory problems, including sleep apnea (interrupted breathing during sleep); and certain cancers. (See Table 9.7.)

Overweight men are more likely to develop cancer of the colon, rectum, and prostate. Overweight women, on the other hand, are at greater risk for developing cancer of the gallbladder, cervix, ovary, uterus, and breast.

Psychological and Social Effects

Despite an increasing amount of research that shows obesity is a very complex medical problem, the obese in American society often suffer discrimination. People sometimes blame the obese for their condition, stereotyping them as lazy and undisciplined. Many think that if overweight people would watch what they eat and get some exercise, they could maintain a normal weight. The obese point out that they suffer job discrimination and are stigmatized by a society that places a great importance on physical appearance, equating attractiveness with being slim.

DIETING

Despite an abundance of diet books, many of which remain on the best-sellers list for many weeks and months, there is no single satisfactory way to achieve long-term weight reduction. The American Dietetic Association reports that in 1998 Americans spent almost $30 billion in the weight-loss industry. Some diets were not very effective; others might have even been harmful.

In one study, a program that supplied a liquid diet combined with pre-portioned foods helped nearly 200 obese adults lose an average of 48 pounds. Three years later, however, only one in eight had kept off 75 percent of the weight, and just over half managed to keep off at least two pounds. Two-fifths had gained back more than they had lost (*University of California at Berkeley Wellness Letter,* Vol. 13, No. 1, October 1996).

Half of Americans are Dieting

DIETERS AND REASONS FOR DIETING. A survey by the Gallup Organization for the Wheat Foods Council (*Setting the Record Straight: What America Thinks About Fad Diets, Nutrition Advice and Food,* Parker, Colo.,

FIGURE 9.3

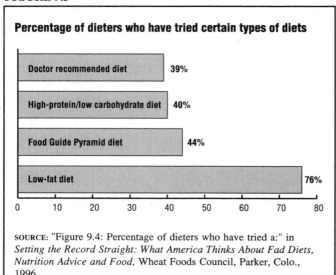

Percentage of dieters who have tried certain types of diets

SOURCE: "Figure 9.4: Percentage of dieters who have tried a:" in *Setting the Record Straight: What America Thinks About Fad Diets, Nutrition Advice and Food,* Wheat Foods Council, Parker, Colo., 1996

FIGURE 9.5

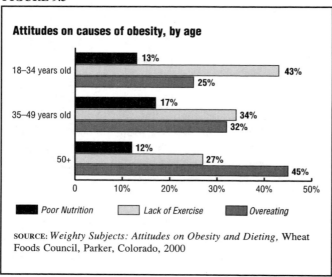

Attitudes on causes of obesity, by age

SOURCE: *Weighty Subjects: Attitudes on Obesity and Dieting,* Wheat Foods Council, Parker, Colorado, 2000

FIGURE 9.4

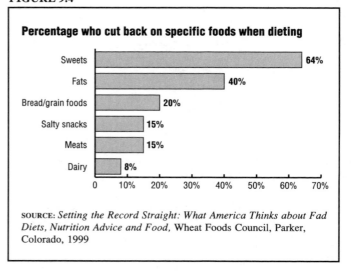

Percentage who cut back on specific foods when dieting

SOURCE: *Setting the Record Straight: What America Thinks about Fad Diets, Nutrition Advice and Food,* Wheat Foods Council, Parker, Colorado, 1999

Food Guide Pyramid, with a foundation of grains, fruits, and vegetables, is the basis of a sensible, healthful eating plan," 40 percent of those same dieters indicated they had tried a high-protein, low-carbohydrate diet.

DIETERS CUT BACK AND ELIMINATE CERTAIN FOODS. Dieters reported cutting back on certain foods—primarily sweets (64 percent of dieters) and fats (40 percent). (See Figure 9.4.) About one-third (32 percent) of dieters reported eliminating certain foods completely from their diets—mainly sweets (62 percent of dieters). Surprisingly, dieters were more likely to stop eating grain foods over fats, salty snacks, meats, or dairy products.

Consumers were split as to the primary cause of obesity. About a third believed overeating was the cause, and a third believed obesity was caused by lack of exercise. Only 14 percent believed poor nutrition to be the cause of obesity. (See Figure 9.5.)

Metabolism

One factor in the battle to lose weight and keep it off is metabolism. Rudolph L. Leibel et al., in "Changes in Energy Expenditure Resulting from Altered Body Weight" (*New England Journal of Medicine,* Vol. 332, No. 10, March 9, 1995), found that the human body has a weight that it naturally gravitates to, whether fat or thin, and it works very hard to maintain that weight. The body adjusts itself to burn calories more slowly if weight is lost below that level and to burn them more quickly if weight is gained above that level.

For example, a 140-pound woman who has lost 10 pounds will burn about 10 to 15 percent fewer calories when she exercises than a woman who maintains that weight effortlessly. Conversely, if a woman has gained 10 pounds, her muscles will burn about 10 to 15 percent more calories to rid her body of the weight.

1999) found that over half (52 percent) of consumers said they had dieted or were currently dieting. Women (59 percent) dieted more often than men (35 percent). (See Figure 9.1.) Adults ages 35 to 49 (60 percent) and those 50 and older (54 percent) were more likely to diet than persons 18 to 34 years old. (See Figure 9.2.) Nearly half of dieters (46 percent) wanted to lose weight, while 16 percent were on a diet to obtain good health, and 11 percent to improve their self-esteem.

DIET PLANS USED. The most popular diet tried by dieters was a low-fat diet (76 percent of dieters), followed by a Food Guide Pyramid eating plan (44 percent). Four in 10 dieters tried a high-protein, low-carbohydrate diet (40 percent) or a diet recommended by their doctors (39 percent). (See Figure 9.3.) Interestingly, although the majority (86 percent) of dieters correctly agreed "the

This study challenged two myths about dieting. The first is that excessive dieting upsets the metabolism and makes it increasingly difficult to lose weight. Metabolism is controlled by the person's weight, not diet. The second myth is that obese people have slow metabolisms. The only people in the study who had sluggish metabolisms were those who were trying to maintain a body weight that was lower than their natural weight. Apparently, however, the body can be reset at a lower weight, as evidenced by those who are successful at weight loss. What that resetting process involves, however, is not yet understood.

Weight Management versus Weight Loss

The National Academy of Sciences has studied weight-loss programs and concluded that program goals need to be changed from "weight loss" to "weight management." Individuals should aim to achieve the best weight possible for good health, not the lowest weight they think they should be. According to the federal guidelines to treat obesity, "the most successful strategies for weight loss include calorie reduction, increased physical activity, and behavior therapy designed to improve eating and physical activity habits."

Characteristics of Successful Dieters

The National Weight Control Registry reveals a number of common characteristics among those who have succeeded in maintaining their weight loss:

- Adherence to a low-calorie, low-fat diet.

- Participation in physical activities.

- Avoidance of diet fads, such as those that limit food intake to certain food groups.

What to Eat?

A major problem with most weight-loss diets is that they are often unscientific and contradictory. Most diet plans are generally written by medical doctors with no formal nutrition training. In the 1970s carbohydrates were declared the cause of obesity, and high-fat, high-protein diets were promoted. Then fats were said to cause obesity, and high-fiber diets became the fad. In the late 1980s, liquid diets were popular. Then, when low fat, high-carbohydrate diets seemed to be the final answer, Americans were told that low-fat, high-carbohydrate foods such as pasta could make them fat. Finally, in the late 1990s, the high-fat, high protein, low-carbohydrate diet of the 1970s made a comeback.

Nutritionists warn against diets that limit the kinds of food a person can eat—for example, those that advise plenty of fats and very little or no carbohydrates. Such diets will likely throw off the body's metabolism. A metabolic disorder called ketosis occurs when, in the absence of carbohydrates, the body burns fats for energy. Compounds related to acetone, called ketones, accumulate in the blood and urine, causing symptoms including nausea, vomiting, bad breath, and lightheadedness. Left untreated, ketosis may lead to dehydration, confusion, or even death.

Fats Are Not Necessarily the Culprits in Obesity

It is believed that the return to a high-fat, high-protein, low carbohydrate diet is an indication of dieters' frustration that low-fat diets have not helped them lose weight. Some dieters think that if a product is labeled "fat-free" or "low-fat," it is all right to eat any quantity of it, regardless of the calories. Often, additional sugar is incorporated in the production of fat-free or low-fat food to make up for the loss of flavor due to the absence or low content of fat; this in turn increases the calorie count. Even if the lower-fat version may not have as many calories as the original product, people may consume more servings of it.

Experts agree that, in the long run, calories count in gaining or losing weight. An excess of calories means weight gain; reduction of calories means weight loss. They believe that the consumption of low-fat and fat-free foods loaded with extra sugars is responsible in part for the increasing weight gain among Americans.

DIET DRUGS

In September 1997 the Food and Drug Administration (FDA) ordered the manufacturers of two diet drugs—fenfluramine, or Pondimin, and dexfenfluramine, commonly known as Redux—to take them off the market after they were linked to potentially fatal damage to the heart valves. Fenfluramine was often used in combination with phentermine, which increased the rate at which calories were burned, and together were popularly called fen-phen. The FDA had approved the two drugs making up fen-phen separately, and doctors could prescribe them in combination with each other.

In the mid-1990s, some people considered fenfluramine and dexfenfluramine miracle pills to combat obesity. The drugs depressed appetite, and were often prescribed with phentermine. Researchers at the University of Rochester Medical School in New York who tested fen-phen reported that dieters who took the drug lost an average of 16 percent of their body weight in 34 weeks, more than three times as much as the control group not taking the diet pills.

In 1996 doctors wrote 18 million prescriptions for Pondimin and Redux, usually in combination with phentermine. Weight-loss clinics mushroomed across the country, many doing business based on these "miracle pills." An estimated 1.2 million to 4.7 million people used the drugs. As of 2001, nearly 2,000 lawsuits are pending against the companies that manufactured Pondimin and Redux.

Other Diet Pills

The latest diet drug to be approved by the FDA is Xenical, whose generic name is orlistat. In April 1999 Xenical was approved for use by patients whose body mass index is 30 (considered obese), as well as for those who are overweight and suffer from high blood pressure, high cholesterol, or diabetes. Xenical does not suppress the appetite like other diet drugs. Instead, it prevents fat absorption by blocking the enzymes that normally break fat down into smaller molecules. Critics charge that, like the recalled drugs fenfluramine and dexfenfluramine, Xenical will be abused as the demand for it increases. The manufacturer of Xenical said that the long-term effects of the drug are not known, nor has the company done any study of the drug's effects on those who want to lose small amounts of weight.

In 1998 the diet drug Meridia was introduced. Its target subjects are similar to Xenical's. Meridia blocks the absorption of serotonin (a brain chemical) into the cells, thus curbing a person's appetite.

EATING DISORDERS

Anorexia Nervosa

Many persons with a weight problem struggle to lose weight and control their overeating. However, some (mainly females but also some males) are obsessed with the fear of gaining weight and literally starve themselves. This condition, known as anorexia nervosa, often begins with a desire to take off a few pounds, and then, experts believe, it becomes an obsession that rules the dieter's life.

Anorexia nervosa results in severe weight loss—to at least 15 percent below normal body weight. Anorexics become terrified of gaining weight and continue to believe they are overweight even though they may be extremely thin. They experience depression and weakness, their nails and hair become brittle, and their skin dries. The medical complications of anorexia are similar to those of starvation. While the body attempts to protect its most vital organs, the heart and brain, it goes into "slow gear." Monthly menstruation stops in women, and breathing, pulse, and thyroid functions slow down. Anemia, swelling joints, and osteoporosis can result. Eventually low blood pressure and an irregular heartbeat may lead to cardiac arrest.

Middle-class, white, teenage girls who strive for perfection, who think they are not "good enough," and who feel controlled by others (parents or peers) are most vulnerable to becoming anorexic. Women whose careers depend on their size—dancers, models, performers, gymnasts—are also at risk for anorexia. Anorexia peaks at age 14 or 15 and again at 18, significant times for stress among young, American women. According to the American Anorexia Bulimia Association, 1 percent of adoles-

cent girls in the United States develop anorexia nervosa, and up to 10 percent of them may die as a result.

Bulimia Nervosa

Also called binge-purge syndrome, bulimia nervosa sometimes, but not always, accompanies anorexia. A bulimic eats compulsively, ingesting huge amounts of high-calorie, high-fat food. Then, disgusted with this behavior, the bulimic purges through forced vomiting and/or abuse of laxatives. The National Institutes of Mental Health (NIMH) estimates that half of people with anorexia will become bulimic.

Many bulimics have normal body weights or are overweight because of the large amounts of food they eat. Unlike persons with binge eating disorders, bulimics purge, fast, or perform vigorous exercises after episodes of binge eating. Bulimics who maintain normal weights can keep their eating disorders a secret for years. The binge-purge cycle can, however, result in heart failure because the body loses vital minerals. The acid in vomit can erode the teeth, glands in the neck can become swollen, and the esophagus can become chronically inflamed.

Some bulimics are addicted to certain foods in the same way alcoholics are addicted to liquor. Many are severely depressed and suicidal. Not all bulimics, however, have psychiatric illnesses. Some bulimic behavior is a "fad," especially on college campuses where overeating and purging are sometimes a part of dorm life. Bulimia peaks in young women between ages 18 and 26. An estimated 3 to 8 percent of women between 12 and 40 are afflicted, although the death rate is unknown.

The NIMH notes that anorexia and bulimia exist primarily in industrialized, economically advanced countries, and that they are much less common among black women. These disorders are almost unheard of in developing or third world countries. "Thinness," it seems, is not highly prized by people whose hunger is not a matter of choice.

Binge Eating Disorder

Binge eating disorder is a newly recognized condition that is believed to affect 2 percent of all adults, or about 1 million to 2 million Americans. It is probably the most common eating disorder. A person with a binge eating disorder frequently eats an abnormally large quantity of food while feeling a loss of control over his or her eating.

Binge eating disorder is common among the obese. Obese persons with the disorder are very likely to have been overweight at younger ages than those without the disorder. They are also more likely to engage in frequent episodes of losing and regaining weight (yo-yo dieting), while also being at risk for the same health problems and diseases that accompany obesity. The disorder is slightly more common in women—three women are affected for every two men. Both whites and blacks are affected by this disorder, although the frequency of occurrence in other ethnic groups is unknown.

EXERCISE

The Exercise-Diet Approach

Some experts are no longer recommending dieting for weight loss but are instead focusing on achieving physical health through exercise. They encourage an appreciation of good food combined with regular exercise.

Steven Blair, director of epidemiology (the study of disease control) and clinical applications at the Cooper Institute for Aerobics Research in Dallas, Texas, has studied over 25,000 men who had received physical fitness tests at the center since 1974. Initially, when Blair compared the health of fat and thin men, he found that fat men were more likely to get sick and die early. But, when Blair entered physical fitness into the equation, he found that it was those who were unfit, regardless of whether they were fat or thin, who were at greatest risk. The diseases common in overweight people were the same as the diseases common in unfit people. Blair claims that earlier studies have linked excess weight and ill health because so many overweight people are sedentary and generally unfit.

Dr. Joann Manson, of the Harvard Medical School, disagrees. She contends that there are very few fit overweight people other than football players. Furthermore, she argues that fat, especially in the area of the belly, contributes to heart disease. Fatty acids are released into the liver, where they interfere with the liver's function of breaking down insulin, increasing the amount of insulin circulating in the body. This sets off a vicious cycle where the cells grow more resistant to metabolizing (burning) fat because of the excess insulin and thereby produce even more liver-damaging fatty acids. This can cause high blood sugar, high blood pressure, and lower levels of HDL, or "good," cholesterol.

Taking a middle position, E. Wayne Callaway, an endocrinologist at George Washington University, thinks that patients who have risk factors, such as high blood pressure or high cholesterol, or who have large stomachs, should make an effort to lose weight. Callaway believes, however, that fat patients who are fit, especially women who have fat in their hips and thighs, should not worry about being overweight.

How Much Exercise Do Americans Need?

Everyone agrees that exercise helps promote good health and weight control. Nonetheless, fitness experts differ as to how much exercise is needed. The Centers for Disease Control and Prevention (CDC) recommends a cumulative 30 minutes or more of moderate exercise over the course of most days. If a person walked for 10 minutes

in the morning, gardened in the afternoon, and took another 10-minute walk after dinner, he or she would get the necessary health benefits of exercise. The CDC estimates that if every sedentary American would engage in some form of moderate exercise for 30 minutes a day, there would be an annual decline in deaths of about 250,000 a year.

The National Institutes of Health (NIH) reports that physical inactivity is a risk factor for heart diseases. Studies have shown that inactive persons are twice as likely to develop heart disease as those who are more active. Even persons who have had heart attacks can improve their chances of survival if they start exercising.

Steven Blair found that men who went from being moderately fit to being highly fit showed a 15 percent decline in mortality. Moreover, when men went from being unfit to moderately fit, there were even greater benefits—a 40 percent decline in deaths from all causes.

Experts stress the importance of exercise for everyone, including the elderly. Studies show that it is never too late to start exercising. In addition, physical activity results in reduced risk of heart disease, disability, and death. Senior citizens who take up weight lifting build their strength, improve their balance, and strengthen their bones, decreasing their risk for osteoporosis. The American College of Sports Medicine suggests that senior citizens engage in aerobic activities for 20 minutes three to five times a week.

What Kind of Exercise Is the Best?

Dr. Kenneth H. Cooper, the head of the Cooper Institute for Aerobics Research, was the first to promote endurance-type exercise, coining the word "aerobics" in 1968 (from *aerobic* meaning "living in air" or "utilizing oxygen"). Examples of aerobic activities are walking, running, biking, and swimming.

While some experts advocate vigorous physical activities, a recent study showed that lightweight activities also benefit the heart. Rozenn N. Lemaitre et al., in "Leisure-Time Physical Activity and the Risk of Primary Cardiac Arrest" (*Archives of Internal Medicine,* Vol. 159, No. 7, April 12, 1999), examined the activities of heart-attack patients ages 25 to 74. The researchers found that, compared to people who did not exercise, those who walked reduced their risk of cardiac arrest by 73 percent. Those who gardened regularly (mowing, raking, pulling weeds) reduced their risk by 66 percent, a similar result achieved by those who performed strenuous exercises (biking, swimming, jogging, tennis, and cross-country and downhill skiing) for a moderate period of time. The walkers in the study spent a median amount of 173 minutes each week; the gardeners, 210 minutes; and those who performed strenuous activities, 50 minutes.

FIGURE 9.6

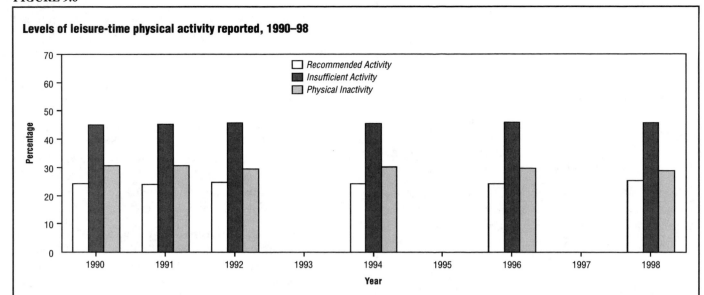

Levels of leisure-time physical activity reported, 1990–98

Note: Recommended level=moderate-intensity activity ≥5 times per week for ≥30 minutes each time, vigorous-intensity ≥3 times per week for ≥20 minutes each time, or both; insufficient=some activity but not enough to be classified as moderate or vigorous; inactive=no leisure-time physical activity during the preceding month. Data were not collected by all states during 1993, 1995, and 1997.

SOURCE: Centers for Disease Control, "Figure 1. Percentage of persons reporting level of leisure-time physical activity, by year--Behavioral Risk Factor Surveillance System, United States, 1990-1998," in *Morbidity and Mortality Weekly Report*, March 9, 2001

LIFESTYLE VERSUS STRUCTURED INTERVENTIONS TO INCREASE PHYSICAL ACTIVITY. Andrea L. Dunn et al. noted that, although a strong link between physical inactivity and ill health has been established, about 60 percent of the U.S. population remains inadequately active or completely inactive. In "Comparison of Lifestyle and Structured Interventions to Increase Physical Activity and Cardiorespiratory Fitness: A Randomized Trial" (*The Journal of the American Medical Association,* Vol. 281, No. 4, January 27, 1999), researchers recognized that many Americans do not exercise for various reasons. These include lack of time, lack of social support, bad weather, lack of access to fitness centers, disruptions of daily routine, and dislike for strenuous physical activity.

With the help of the Cooper Institute Institutional Review Board in Dallas, Texas, researchers compared the effects on sedentary adults of improving physical activity and cardiorespiratory fitness, using two intervention programs—a physical activity program geared toward a person's lifestyle versus a traditional fitness center-based program. Participants in the lifestyle group were advised to perform at least 30 minutes of moderate-intensive physical activity on most or all days of the week in a manner suited to their lifestyle. During regular meetings, they learned cognitive and behavioral strategies to maintain their physical activity. Group meetings involved mall walking, volleyball, and other activities to reinforce their cognitive and behavioral skills. The study showed that at 24 months, participants of both the lifestyle group and

FIGURE 9.7

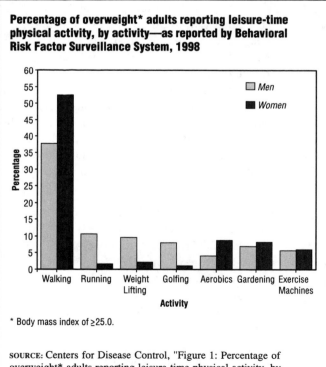

Percentage of overweight* adults reporting leisure-time physical activity, by activity—as reported by Behavioral Risk Factor Surveillance System, 1998

* Body mass index of ≥25.0.

SOURCE: Centers for Disease Control, "Figure 1: Percentage of overweight* adults reporting leisure-time physical activity, by activity--United States, Behavioral Risk Factor Surveillance System, 1998," in *Morbidity and Mortality Weekly Report*, April 21, 2000

TABLE 9.8

Leisure-time physical activity patterns among overweight adults trying to lose weight, by selected characteristics—as reported in Behavioral Risk Factor Surveillance System, 1998

Characteristic	Men					Women				
	Sample size	% using physical activity to lose weight	(95% CI[1])	% meeting physical activity guidelines[2]	(95%CI[1])	Sample size	% using physical activity to lose weight	(95% CI[1])	% meeting physical activity guidelines[2]	(95% CI[1])
Age (yrs)										
18–24	903	83.8	(80.3–87.3)	25.7	(21.6–29.8)	1,294	77.5	(73.4–81.6)	20.3	(16.8–23.8)
25–34	2,570	76.7	(74.4–79.1)	22.5	(20.0–25.1)	3,790	72.0	(69.8–74.2)	20.4	(18.4–22.4)
35–44	3,685	68.2	(65.7–70.8)	18.8	(16.8–20.8)	5,173	65.5	(63.3–67.7)	18.6	(16.8–20.4)
45–54	3,499	63.0	(60.5–65.6)	21.0	(18.8–23.2)	4,391	62.1	(59.8–64.5)	18.4	(16.6–20.2)
55–64	2,256	57.2	(54.1–60.3)	23.8	(21.1–26.5)	3,183	55.4	(52.7–58.1)	18.3	(16.1–20.5)
≥ 65	2,120	55.1	(51.8–58.4)	25.5	(22.6–28.4)	3,734	46.7	(44.2–49.3)	18.7	(16.5–20.9)
Race/Ethnicity[3]										
White	12,426	66.5	(65.3–67.7)	22.8	(21.6–24.0)	16,622	63.5	(62.3–64.7)	20.1	(19.1–21.1)
Black	1,049	70.1	(66.2–74.0)	22.6	(18.9–26.3)	2,687	62.8	(60.1–65.5)	16.9	(14.6–19.3)
Hispanic	1,017	63.8	(59.1–68.5)	17.1	(13.6–20.6)	1,614	52.7	(48.8–56.6)	14.3	(11.8–16.9)
Other	541	68.4	(60.6–76.2)	23.0	(15.6–30.5)	642	63.5	(55.7–71.3)	20.6	(14.7–26.5)
Education level										
Less than high school	1,575	47.4	(43.3–51.5)	17.7	(14.4–21.0)	2,921	44.6	(41.7–47.5)	12.7	(10.7–14.7)
High school graduate	4,327	65.7	(63.5–67.9)	19.9	(18.1–21.7)	7,811	60.6	(58.8–62.4)	17.4	(16.0–18.8)
Some college	4,018	68.5	(66.3–70.7)	22.5	(20.5–24.5)	6,234	66.2	(64.2–68.2)	21.0	(19.4–22.6)
College graduate	5,113	72.7	(70.7–74.7)	25.5	(23.5–27.5)	4,599	71.9	(69.9–73.9)	23.5	(21.5–25.5)
Region[4]										
Northeast	2,939	68.9	(66.2–71.6)	23.0	(20.5–25.6)	3,777	62.0	(59.5–64.6)	18.4	(16.2–20.6)
Midwest	2,365	69.7	(67.2–72.3)	24.6	(22.3–27.0)	3,593	64.1	(61.9–66.3)	18.3	(16.7–19.9)
South	4,060	62.0	(60.0–64.0)	20.1	(18.5–21.7)	6,518	59.2	(57.6–60.8)	17.8	(16.4–19.2)
West	5,669	67.1	(64.8–69.5)	21.9	(19.9–23.9)	7,677	63.6	(61.4–65.8)	20.8	(19.2–22.4)
BMI status[5]										
Overweight	8,729	69.7	(68.1–71.3)	24.5	(23.1–25.9)	12,042	66.2	(64.8–67.6)	21.3	(20.1–22.5)
Obese	6,304	62.3	(60.5–64.1)	18.8	(17.2–20.4)	9,523	57.1	(55.5–58.7)	16.1	(14.9–17.3)
Total	**15,033**	**66.6**	**(65.4–67.8)**	**22.2**	**(21.2–23.2)**	**21,565**	**62.2**	**(61.2–63.2)**	**19.0**	**(18.2–19.8)**

[1] Confidence interval.

[2] Five or more times per week and ≥ 30 minutes per session.

[3] Racial groups other than white, black, and Hispanic were combined because, when analyzed separately, data were too small for meaningful analysis.

[4] Northeast=Connecticut, Maine, Massachusetts, New Hampshire, New Jersey, New York, Pennsylvania, Rhode Island, and Vermont; Midwest=Illinois, Indiana, Iowa, Kansas, Michigan, Minnesota, Missouri, Nebraska, North Dakota, Ohio, South Dakota, and Wisconsin; South=Alabama, Arkansas, Delaware, District of Columbia, Florida, Georgia, Kentucky, Louisiana, Maryland, Mississippi, North Carolina, Oklahoma, South Carolina, Tennessee, Texas, Virginia, and West Virginia; and West=Arizona, California, Colorado, Hawaii, Idaho, Montana, Nevada, New Mexico, Oregon, Utah, Washington, and Wyoming.

[5] Body mass index (BMI) of 25.0–29.9 for overweight persons and ≥ 30.0 for obese persons.

SOURCE: Centers for Disease Control, "Table 1: Leisure-time physical activity patterns among overweight adults trying to lose weight, by selected characteristics--United States, Behavioral Risk Factor Surveillance System, 1998" in *Morbidity and Mortality Weekly Report*, April 21, 2000

the fitness center-based intervention improved their physical activity, cardiorespiratory fitness, and blood pressure, and achieved positive changes to their percentage of body fat.

How Much Do Americans Exercise?

The CDC, in their *Morbidity and Mortality Weekly Report* (March 2001), found that most adults are not getting enough physical activity. About 50 percent got insufficient physical activity (some activity but not enough to be classified as moderate or vigorous). One-third (30 percent) were physically inactive, and only 25 percent followed recommendations and underwent moderate to intense activity five or more times per week for 30 minutes each time or vigorous activity three or more times each week for 20 or more minutes each time. (See Figure 9.6.)

The CDC also studied physical activity among overweight adults trying to lose weight. Results were presented in the April 2000 issue of *The Morbidity and Mortality Weekly Report*. The majority of overweight adults (over 50 percent of women and about 38 percent of men) reported walking for physical activity. Far fewer (10 percent or less) chose other activities—running, weight lifting, golfing, aerobics, gardening, or exercise machines. (See Figure 9.7.)

Among both men and women, younger and more educated people were more likely to use physical activity to lose weight and to meet their physical activity requirements. (See Table 9.8.)

THE SURGEON GENERAL'S REPORT. The report of the Surgeon General, *Physical Activity and Health* (CDC and the President's Council on Physical Fitness and Sports,

Washington, D.C., 1996), stated that only about 15 percent of adults participated in regular (three times a week for at least 20 minutes) vigorous physical activity. Approximately 22 percent of adults engaged in any level of physical activity for a sustained period of time (five times a week for at least 30 minutes). About 25 percent did no physical exercise at all.

Inactivity was more prevalent among women than men, among blacks and Hispanics than whites, among older than younger adults, and among the less wealthy than the more wealthy. The most popular activities were walking and gardening, or yard work.

About one-half of young people ages 12 to 21 participated in regular vigorous activity; one-fourth were not active at all. Inactivity was more likely in young females than in young males and in black young females than in white young females. Physical activity declined sharply as the grade in school increased. Only 19 percent of high school students reported being physically active for 20 minutes or more in daily physical education classes.

CHAPTER 10
HUNGER AND PUBLIC ASSISTANCE PROGRAMS

In the early 1800s Thomas Robert Malthus, a British economist and mathematician, developed the theory that the food supply grows arithmetically, increasing by two, four, six, eight, ten, etc., but that population grows geometrically—two, four, eight, sixteen, thirty-two, etc. Based on this theory, Malthus believed the world would eventually run out of food, and people would face starvation and death.

Thomas Malthus could not have imagined the spectacular developments in the science of growing and preserving food. With modern technology, farmers have been able to produce more food per acre than ever before. Two hundred years ago, fresh food could not be moved from one region to another without spoiling because there was no refrigeration, and transportation was very slow. Today food can be shipped around the world and eaten almost as fresh as it was when first picked, caught, or prepared.

Medical knowledge and technology, however, are keeping people alive longer and longer, and this combined with the fact that the population of developing countries continues to increase, means that some observers again fear that food supplies will not be enough to feed everyone in the world.

MOST AMERICANS ARE WELL FED

One measure of the wealth of a country is the amount of grain it uses per capita (per person). In some developing countries, the average person consumes about 400 pounds a year, leaving very little grain for animals that are being raised for food.

The typical North American usually uses 2000 pounds of grain—one ton—each a year. Of this ton, less than 200 pounds is eaten directly in the form of bread, pasta, or breakfast cereal. The largest portion goes to feed livestock and is indirectly eaten in the form of meat, milk, and eggs. The average North American consumes up to

five times as many agricultural resources as the average citizen of Nigeria, India, or Bangladesh.

IS THERE HUNGER IN AMERICA?

Hunger and Food Insecurity

Even though the United States is one of the richest countries in the world, some Americans are still poor and hungry. According to the U.S. Department of Agriculture (USDA),

> "Hunger" is the uneasy or painful sensation caused by a lack of food. It can result from the recurrent and involuntary lack of access to food. "Severe hunger" exists in households when children go hungry or adults experience prolonged or acute hunger. "Food insecurity" is used to describe inadequate access to enough food at all times for a healthy, active life. It can be a warning sign for hunger.

The latest USDA survey of hunger and food insecurity, conducted in 1999 (a year considered economically strong), found that the large majority of Americans (91.3 percent) were food secure, up from 89.7 percent in 1995. (See Table 10.1.) About 8.7 percent of all U.S. households (31 million Americans) reported experiencing food insecurity due to a lack of financial resources, down from 10.3 percent in 1995.

Characteristics of Low-Income, Food-Insecure Households

Approximately 32.3 percent of low-income U.S. households (those with incomes below 130 percent of the poverty level) reported being food insecure—concerned about the adequacy of their food supply. Not all food-insecure households equally experienced hunger. About 10.7 percent of these households reported experiencing hunger; this figure rose to 12.9 percent for female-head, no-spouse households, and 13.7 percent for men living alone. Black (13.1 percent) and Hispanic (10.8 percent)

TABLE 10.1

Prevalence of food security, food insecurity, and hunger for households and persons, by year (adjusted for cross-year comparability)

Category	Total* 1,000	Food secure 1,000	Food secure Percent	Food insecure: All 1,000	Food insecure: All Percent	Food insecure: Without hunger 1,000	Food insecure: Without hunger Percent	Food insecure: With hunger 1,000	Food insecure: With hunger Percent
Households									
1995	100,445	90,097	89.7	10,348	10.3	6,402	6.4	3,946	3.9
1996	101,508	90,964	89.6	10,544	10.4	6,407	6.3	4,137	4.1
1997	102,373	93,459	91.3	8,914	8.7	5,760	5.6	3,154	3.1
1998	103,480	92,972	89.8	10,509	10.2	6,820	6.6	3,689	3.6
1999	104,816	95,664	91.3	9,152	8.7	6,166	5.9	2,987	2.8
All persons in households									
1995	261,342	230,910	88.4	30,431	11.6	19,742	7.6	10,689	4.1
1996	264,780	233,221	88.1	31,559	11.9	20,119	7.6	11,440	4.3
1997	266,128	240,009	90.2	26,120	9.8	18,045	6.8	8,075	3.0
1998	268,886	237,721	88.4	31,165	11.6	21,771	8.1	9,394	3.5
1999	270,609	243,652	90.0	26,957	10.0	19,441	7.2	7,515	2.8
Adults in households									
1995	191,063	172,862	90.5	18,200	9.5	11,611	6.1	6,589	3.4
1996	193,608	175,003	90.4	18,606	9.6	11,582	6.0	7,024	3.6
1997	195,180	179,420	91.9	15,761	8.1	10,601	5.4	5,160	2.6
1998	197,423	178,631	90.5	18,792	9.5	12,657	6.4	6,135	3.1
1999	199,116	182,793	91.8	16,323	8.2	11,447	5.8	4,875	2.4
Children in households									
1995	70,279	58,048	82.6	12,231	17.4	8,131	11.6	4,100	5.8
1996	71,172	58,218	81.8	12,953	18.2	8,537	12.0	4,416	6.2
1997	70,948	60,589	85.4	10,359	14.6	7,444	10.5	2,915	4.1
1998	71,463	59,090	82.7	12,373	17.3	9,114	12.8	3,259	4.6
1999	71,493	60,859	85.1	10,634	14.9	7,994	11.2	2,640	3.7

SOURCE: Andrews, Margaret et al, "Table 1: Prevalence of food security, food insecurity, and hunger for households and persons, by year," in *Household Food Security in the U.S., 1999*, USDA Food Assistance and Nutrition Research Report No. 8, U.S. Department of Agriculture, Economic Research Service, Food and Rural Economics Division

low-income households were more likely than their white counterparts (9.5 percent) to go hungry. (See Table 10.2.)

FEDERAL PROGRAMS THAT FEED THE HUNGRY

Food-assistance programs were begun during the Great Depression of the 1930s to help feed the poor and the unemployed, and to keep farm prices stable by giving the surplus (more food than could be profitably sold on the market) to people who needed it. Established in 1969, the USDA's Food and Nutrition Service (FNS) administers the nation's current food-assistance programs. The agency's goals are to provide needy people with access to a more nutritious diet, to improve the eating habits of the nation's children, and to help farmers by stabilizing farm prices through the purchase and distribution of surplus foods.

The FNS works in partnership with the states in all its programs. States determine most administrative details regarding distribution of food benefits and eligibility of participants, and the FNS provides funding to cover most of the states' administrative costs. In fiscal year 1998 (October 1, 1997 through September 30, 1998), the federal government spent $33.7 billion in food-assistance programs. (See Table 10.3.) The amount spent in fiscal year (FY) 1998 was a 6 percent drop from the previous FY, when $35.8 billion was spent.

In general, food assistance expenditures follow macroeconomic conditions, that is, when unemployment is high, food assistance expenditures are relatively high and vice versa. (See Figure 10.1.) Note that dollars spent have been inflation-adjusted to produce "real" food assistance expenditures.

Food Stamp Program

The Food Stamp Program, the largest of the federal food-assistance programs, began as a pilot program in 1961. Congress established it as a permanent program through the Food Stamp Act of 1964 (PL 88-525). It is designed to increase the food-purchasing ability of low-income families to the point where they can afford nutritionally adequate low-cost diets. Paper coupons or electronic benefits transfers (EBTs) are used in place of money in food stores all over the country. Food stamps are good only for foods to prepare at home and not for tobacco, alcohol, lunch-counter items, or foods to be eaten in the store.

In order to be eligible for food stamps, individuals must meet income guidelines and certain work requirements.

TABLE 10.2

Prevalence of food security, food insecurity, and hunger in households with income below 130 percent of the poverty line, 1999
(Based on unadjusted data)

| | Total[1] | Food secure | | Food insecure: | | | | | |
| | | | | All | | Without hunger | | With hunger | |
Category	1,000	1,000	Percent	1,000	Percent	1,000	Percent	1,000	Percent
All low-income households	17,432	11,799	67.7	5,633	32.3	3,767	21.6	1,866	10.7
Persons in low-income households	47,159	30,283	64.2	16,876	35.8	12,064	25.6	4,812	10.2
Adults in low-income households	29,684	20,073	67.6	9,611	32.4	6,686	22.5	2,925	9.9
Children in low-income households	17,475	10,210	58.4	7,265	41.6	5,378	30.8	1,888	10.8
Household composition:									
With children < 6	4,070	2,475	60.8	1,595	39.2	1,234	30.3	361	8.9
With children < 18	7,583	4,525	59.7	3,058	40.3	2,278	30.0	780	10.3
Married couple families	3,022	1,919	63.5	1,103	36.5	880	29.1	223	7.4
Female head, no spouse	3,896	2,172	55.7	1,724	44.3	1,224	31.4	500	12.9
Male head, no spouse	515	329	64.0	185	36.0	146	28.3	40	7.7
Other household with child[2]	150	105	70.1	45	29.9	28	18.5	17	11.4
With no children < 18	9,849	7,274	73.9	2,575	26.1	1,489	15.1	1,086	11.0
More than one adult	3,780	2,878	76.2	902	23.8	534	14.1	367	9.7
Women living alone	3,953	2,963	75.0	990	25.0	561	14.2	429	10.9
Men living alone	2,116	1,433	67.7	683	32.3	394	18.6	289	13.7
Households with elderly	4,299	3,518	81.8	781	18.2	527	12.3	255	5.9
Elderly living alone	2,577	2,147	83.3	431	16.7	266	10.3	165	6.4
Race/ethnicity of households:									
White non-Hispanic	9,352	6,855	73.3	2,496	26.7	1,607	17.2	889	9.5
Black non-Hispanic	4,082	2,435	59.6	1,648	40.4	1,112	27.2	535	13.1
Hispanic[3]	3,221	1,974	61.3	1,247	38.7	900	27.9	347	10.8
Other non-Hispanic	776	535	68.9	242	31.1	147	18.9	95	12.2
Area of residence:									
Inside metropolitan area	12,978	8,602	66.3	4,376	33.7	2,902	22.4	1,473	11.3
In central city[4]	5,824	3,677	63.1	2,147	36.9	1,439	24.7	708	12.2
Not in central city[4]	4,536	3,097	68.3	1,438	31.7	956	21.1	482	10.6
Outside metropolitan area	4,454	3,197	71.8	1,257	28.2	864	19.4	393	8.8
Census geographic region:									
Northeast	2,756	1,939	70.3	817	29.7	540	19.6	277	10.1
Midwest	3,386	2,399	70.8	988	29.2	674	19.9	314	9.3
South	7,390	4,966	67.2	2,424	32.8	1,666	22.5	758	10.3
West	3,899	2,496	64.0	1,403	36.0	887	22.7	517	13.3

Notes to tables
[1]Total households in each category exclude households whose food security status is unknown. These households did not give a valid response to any of the questions in the food security scale, and they gave no indication of food security on preliminary screening questions. In 1999 these households represented 348,000 households (0.3 percent of all households). However, some of these households were screened out and deemed food secure under the common screen, reducing the missing households in table 1 to 216,000 (0.2 percent of all households) and raising the number of households with valid responses to 104,816,000.
[2]Households with children in complex living arrangements, e.g., children of other relatives or unrelated roommate or border.
[3]Hispanics may be of any race.
[4]Subtotals do not add to metropolitan totals because central-city residence is not identified for about 17 percent of households in metropolitan statistical areas.

SOURCE: Margaret Andrews et al, "Table 3--1999: Prevalence of food security, food insecurity, and hunger in households with income below 130 percent of the poverty line, by selected characteristics of households," in *Household Food Security in the U.S., 1999*, USDA Food Assistance and Nutrition Research Report No. 8, U.S. Department of Agriculture, Economic Research Service, Food and Rural Economics Division

Benefits are based on household size, income, and certain nonfood expenses (including housing costs, dependent-care expenses, and child-support payments) and are adjusted annually for inflation. Generally, the monthly income of the household must be at or below 130 percent of the federal poverty guidelines. In FY 1998 monthly benefits averaged $71 a person or about $170 per household.

After an all-time peak monthly participation of 28 million people in the spring of 1994, food stamp enrollment declined continuously, down to 22.9 million recipients in FY 1997. In fact, the Food Stamp Program accounted for much of the decrease (-7.1 percent) in total food-assistance expenditures for the first half of 1999. (See Table 10.3.)

The decline in participation was due in part to the changes brought about by the 1996 Personal Responsibility and Work Opportunity Reconciliation Act (PL 104-193; also called the welfare-reform law), which eliminated benefits to most legal immigrants and able-bodied adults with no dependents. (In 1998 the Agricultural Research, Extension, and Education Reform Act [PL 105-185] restored food stamp benefits to immigrants who were receiving benefits or assistance for blindness or disability, were younger than 18, or were age 65 or older as of August 22, 1996). The continuing strong economy and

TABLE 10.3

Food assistance program outlays, fiscal year 1998 and the first half of fiscal year 1999

| Program | Fiscal 1998 expenditures | | First half of fiscal 1999 expenditures[1] | |
| | Total | October-March | October-March | Change from first half of fiscal 1998 |
	Million dollars	Million dollars	Million dollars	Percent
Food stamp-related programs	**20,130.5**	**10,326.3**	**9,647.5**	**-6.6**
Food Stamp Program[2]	18,916.1	9,719.1	9,024.3	-7.1
Nutrition Assistance Programs[2]	1,214.4	607.2	623.2	2.6
Child nutrition programs[3]	**9,049.8**	**5,189.2**	**5,324.0**	**2.6**
National School Lunch	5,828.3	3,586.0	3,673.0	2.4
School Breakfast	1,271.2	769.0	795.7	3.5
Child and Adult Care[2]	1,552.1	779.4	802.1	2.9
Summer Food Service[2]	261.5	4.9	4.2	-14.3
Special Milk	17.0	9.2	9.0	-2.2
Supplemental food programs	**3,983.3**	**1,930.2**	**1,989.1**	**3.1**
WIC[2]	3,890.0	1,883.2	1,938.7	2.9
Commodity Supplemental Food Program[2]	93.3	47.0	50.4	7.2
Food donation programs	**457.4**	**206.1**	**218.8**	**6.2**
Food Distribution on Indian Reservations[2]	71.6	34.3	35.9	4.7
Nutrition Program for the Elderly	141.1	69.4	68.6	-1.2
Disaster Feeding	.3	.1	.5	400.0
TEFAP	235.1	100.9	110.7	9.7
Charitable Institutions and Summer Camps	9.2	1.4	2.9	107.1
All programs[4]	**33,728.5**	**17,702.5**	**17,228.7**	**-2.7**

[1]Data are reported as of March 1999 and are subject to revision.
[2]Includes administrative expenses.
[3]Total includes the Federal share of State administration expenses.
[4]Total includes Federal food program administration expenses.

SOURCE: Victor Oliveira, "Table 1: Food Assistance Program Outlays Continue to Decline in First Half of Fiscal 1999," in "Domestic Food Assistance Expenditures Drop Again," *Food Review*, vol. 22, issue 3, Sept-Dec, 1999.

the accompanying decrease in unemployment also contributed to the decline.

PARTICIPATION IN THE FOOD STAMP PROGRAM. The FY 1998 survey of the characteristics of food stamp households found that half (51 percent) were children, 39 percent were non-elderly adults, and 8 percent were elderly. More than 15 percent were elderly or disabled. Single-parent households with children accounted for 39.6 percent of participating households, while elderly persons who lived alone made up another 14.4 percent. Of the total recipients, whites comprised 40 percent; African Americans, 36.3 percent; and Hispanics, 18.3 percent. Over a third of participating households were very poor, with monthly incomes below half the federal income poverty guidelines.

ELECTRONIC BENEFITS TRANSFER (EBT). In the past, food stamp participants received their monthly benefits in the form of paper coupons to redeem for foods at authorized food stores. In an effort to eliminate illegal trafficking in food stamps, the government introduced a system of electronic benefits transfer (EBT), which operates like a bank card. When food purchases are made, the store uses the card to debit the recipient's food stamp account. In 1998 about 40 percent of food stamp benefits were delivered using EBT, and that percentage will continue to grow.

Child Nutrition Programs

The USDA operates five programs to provide meals and snacks to preschool and school age children. In 1998 federal expenditures for these programs totaled $9 billion, a 4 percent increase from 1997. (See Table 10.3.) This is a continuation of the trend of steady increase in program costs, which have grown 82 percent over the past 12 years.

NATIONAL SCHOOL LUNCH PROGRAM. The National School Lunch Program provides lunch to children in public and nonprofit private schools and in residential child care institutions. The USDA provides cash and some commodities to these schools to offset food-service costs. In return, the schools must serve lunches that meet federal nutritional requirements. The program is available to virtually every child, and low-income students may qualify to receive their lunches free or at a reduced price.

The cost of the National School Lunch Program has been rising steadily for many years. It is the second largest food-assistance program. In 1998 over 26 million children in almost 93,000 schools and residential child

FIGURE 10.1

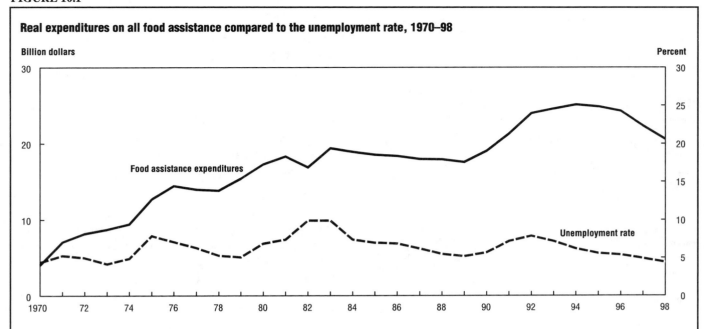

Real expenditures on all food assistance compared to the unemployment rate, 1970–98

SOURCE: Craig Gunderson et al, "Figure 5: U.S. real expenditures on food assistance expenditures and the unemployment rate, 1970–98," in *A Comparison of Food Assistance Programs in Mexico and the U.S.*, Food Assistance and Nutrition Research Report No. 6, Economic Research Service, U.S. Department of Agriculture, 2000

care institutions received subsidized lunches at a cost of $5.8 billion. (See Table 10.3.) Almost 50 percent of the children got free lunches, and another 8 percent received reduced-priced lunches.

A 1992 *School Nutrition Dietary Assessment* found that although school lunches were nutritious, they provided 38 percent of calories from total fat and 15 percent of calories from saturated fat. This is more than the recommendations by the USDA *Dietary Guidelines for Americans* that 30 percent or less of calories come from total fat and less than 10 percent of calories come from saturated fat. The study also found that lunches provided an average of 1,479 milligrams of sodium—almost two-thirds the National Research Council's recommendation for daily intake.

Starting in the 1996-97 school year, schools had to meet USDA nutritional guidelines in promoting the health of children. School cafeterias have always had the difficult task of trying to serve nutritious meals to children who often prefer high-fat, high-sodium meals like pizza or macaroni and cheese. The USDA's Team Nutrition Program is helping school cafeterias make changes to their menus, reducing the fat content of foods and providing more healthy choices.

SCHOOL BREAKFAST PROGRAM. Begun in 1966, the School Breakfast Program became permanent in 1975. Eligibility is the same as for the National School Lunch Program. Although it has grown steadily over the past two years, the breakfast program is still smaller than the lunch program. In recent years, the USDA has encouraged schools that participate in the lunch program to offer the School Breakfast Program.

In FY 1998 the program served almost 1.2 billion breakfasts to low-income children at a cost of $1.27 billion. (See Table 10.3.) Approximately 80 percent of the meals were served free, and another 6 percent were offered at reduced prices.

CHILD AND ADULT CARE FOOD PROGRAM. The Child and Adult Care Food Program provides cash and food to child care centers, family day care homes, and adult day care centers. In FY 1997, 1.6 billion meals were served—98 percent in child care centers and family day care homes and 2 percent in adult day care centers. Expenditures decreased 1.2 percent, from $1.57 billion in 1997 to $1.55 billion in 1998. (See Table 10.3.) Over 80 percent of all meals were free; another 4 percent were at reduced prices.

SUMMER FOOD SERVICE PROGRAM. During school vacations, the Summer Food Service Program provides free meals and snacks to children 18 years and younger and to handicapped persons over age 18 in places where at least half of the children come from households with incomes at or below 185 percent of the federal income poverty guidelines. In FY 1998 over 133 million meals and snacks were served, totaling $261.5 million in expenditures. (See Table 10.3.)

TABLE 10.4

Distribution of WIC participants by category, 1992–98

Distribution of WIC Participants by Participant Category in 1996 and 1998

Participant Category	Number of Participants 1996	Numbers of Participants 1998	Percent Change 1996-1998
Women			
Pregnant women	877,747	892,674	+1.7%
Breastfeeding women	330,176	389,391	+17.9
Postpartum women	567,913	591,049	+4.1
Total women	1,775,837	1,873,115	+5.5
Infants	1,988,789	2,048,625	+3.0
Children	3,982,815	4,121,016	+3.5
US WIC	7,747,441	8,042,758	3.8

Distribution of WIC Participants by Participant Category 1992, 1994, 1996, 1998

Participant Category	Percent of Total WIC Participants			
	1992	1994	1996	1998
Women				
Pregnant women	13.6%	12.0%	11.3%	11.1%
Breastfeeding women	3.6	4.0	4.3	4.8
Postpartum women	5.2	7.2	7.3	7.3
Total women	22.4	23.1	22.9	23.3
Infants	30.1	26.9	25.7	25.5
Children	47.5	50.2	51.4	51.2
US WIC	5,754,003	6,907,849	7,747,441	8,042,758

Note: For the biennial PC reports, participants are defined as persons on WIC master lists who are certified to receive WIC benefits in April 1998, including individuals who do not claim or use their food instruments. This differs from FNS administrative data in which participants are defined as individuals who pick up or redeem their food vouchers.

SOURCE: "Exhibit 2.1," in *WIC Participation and Program Characteristics 1998*, Report WIC-00-PC, U.S. Department of Agriculture, Food and Nutrition Service, May 2000

SPECIAL MILK PROGRAM. Expansion of the National School Lunch and School Breakfast Programs, which include subsidized milk, has led to a substantial reduction in the Special Milk Program since its peak in the late 1960s. Participation is now limited to schools, summer camps, and child care institutions that have no federally assisted meal program, or to prekindergarten or kindergarten children who attend half-day sessions and have no access to milk programs. Milk is offered free or at reduced cost. In FY 1998 the program cost $17 million, a slight decrease over the previous year. (See Table 10.3.)

Supplemental Food Programs

SPECIAL SUPPLEMENTAL NUTRITION PROGRAM FOR WOMEN, INFANTS, AND CHILDREN (WIC). The Special Supplemental Nutrition Program for Women, Infants, and Children (WIC) is the third largest food-assistance program. It provides nutritious supplemental foods, nutrition education, and health care referrals at no cost to low-income pregnant and postpartum (period after childbirth) women, infants, and children up to the age of five. To be eligible, income must be below 185 percent of the federal income poverty guidelines. States can, however, set lower income limits.

Although all food-assistance programs promote improved nutrition as an objective, only WIC requires that a health official or a nutritionist first determine a recipient's nutritional needs. Eligible mothers get monthly food vouchers, or coupons, from their local health clinics. They can redeem these vouchers for specific foods rich in nutrients, such as infant formula, eggs, fruit juice, milk, cheese, and cereal. In FY 1997 these monthly benefits averaged $31.68 per person.

Under the WIC Farmers' Market Nutrition Program, recipients receive coupons to buy fresh fruits and vegetables at participating farmers' markets. A study sponsored by the USDA Food and Nutrition Service in 1990 showed that women who participated in the program during their pregnancies had lower Medicaid (government-paid health care for lower-income people) costs for themselves and their babies than women who did not participate.

Participation in WIC continues to grow, with expenditures totaling $3.9 billion in FY 1998, a 2.6 percent increase from 1997. (See Table 10.3.) In 1998, 8 million persons received WIC. (See Table 10.4.) About half of WIC recipients are children and one-quarter are infants.

COMMODITY SUPPLEMENTAL FOOD PROGRAM (CSFP). The Commodity Supplemental Food Program (CSFP) serves women and children up to six years who are not WIC participants, as well as low-income people age 60 and over. While WIC uses vouchers, the CSFP distributes monthly food parcels. In FY 1997 the program provided monthly food parcels to about 370,000 people. As more women and children switch to the WIC program, the CSFP serves an increasing proportion of the elderly. In FY 1997 the elderly accounted for nearly two-thirds of all participants, an increase of 11 percent from the previous year. Costs fell 5.4 percent, from $98.7 million in 1997 to $93.3 million in 1998. (See Table 10.3.)

Food Donation Programs

FOOD DISTRIBUTION PROGRAM ON INDIAN RESERVATIONS. The USDA provides food to families who live on or near Indian reservations. The program is an alternative to the Food Stamp Program for those whose remote location limits access to food stores. In 1998 about 124,000 Native Americans participated in the program. Expenditures for this program in FY 1998 were $71.6 million. (See Table 10.3.)

NUTRITION PROGRAM FOR THE ELDERLY. The Nutrition Program for the Elderly provides cash and food to the states for meals for senior citizens. Food is served in senior-citizen centers or delivered by Meals-on-Wheels programs. There is no income test for eligibility; all persons over 60 years of age are eligible. Recipients can contribute as much as they wish to the cost of the meals, although the meals are free to those who cannot afford to pay. In 1998 the program served 247 million meals at a cost of $141.1 million, down 2.8 percent from 1997. (See Table 10.3.)

THE EMERGENCY FOOD ASSISTANCE PROGRAM (TEFAP). The Emergency Food Assistance Program (TEFAP) was started in 1982 to help distribute government surpluses of butter, cheese, nonfat dry milk, honey, rice, cornmeal, and flour to needy families. Federal costs for TEFAP rapidly increased until the late 1980s, when government surpluses were used up. As these government stocks were depleted, food distribution had to be either discontinued or financed through appropriated (Congress-approved) funds.

The Federal Agriculture Improvement and Reform Act (PL 104-127; also called the 1996 farm bill) made TEFAP a permanent program based on funding rather than purchases of surplus foods. In FY 1997 the TEFAP and the Food Donation Programs to Soup Kitchens and Food Banks were combined into a single program, and in 1998 expenditures totaled nearly $235 million. (See Table 10.3.)

IMPORTANT NAMES AND ADDRESSES

American Dietetic Association
16 West Jackson Blvd.
Chicago, IL 60606
(312) 899-0040
FAX: (312) 899-4899
URL: http://www.eatright.org

Council for Responsible Nutrition
1875 Eye St. NW, Suite 400
Washington, DC 20006-5409
(202) 872-1488
FAX: (202) 872-9594
E-mail: webmaster@crnusa.org
URL: http://www.crnusa.org

Environmental Working Group
1718 Connecticut Ave. NW, Suite 600
Washington, DC 20009
(202) 667-6982
FAX: (202) 232-2592
E-mail: info@ewg.org
URL: http://www.ewg.org

Food Marketing Institute
655 15th Street NW
Washington, DC 20005
(202) 452-8444
FAX: (202) 429-4519
E-mail: fmi@fmi.org
URL: http://www.fmi.org

National Center for Food and Agricultural Policy
1616 P St. NW, 1st Floor
Washington, DC 20036
(202) 328-5048
FAX: (202) 328-5133
E-mail: stovall@ncfap.org
URL: http://www.ncfap.org

National Restaurant Association
1200 17th St. NW
Washington, DC 20036-3097
(202) 331-5900

FAX: (202) 331-2429
E-mail: info@dineout.org
URL: http://www.restaurant.org

Public Citizen
Health Research Group
1600 20th St. NW
Washington, DC 20009
(202) 588-1000
FAX: (202) 588-7796
URL: http://www.citizen.org

U.S. Department of Agriculture
Agricultural Research Service
14th & Independence Ave. SW
Room 302A
Washington, DC 20250-0300
(202) 720-3656
FAX: (202) 720-5427
E-mail: arsweb@nal.usda.gov
URL: http://www.ars.usda.gov

U.S. Department of Agriculture
Center for Nutrition Policy and Promotion
1120 20th St. NW
Suite 200 North Lobby
Washington, DC 20036
(202) 418-2312
E-mail: cnpp-web@www.usda.gov
URL: http://www.usda.gov/cnpp

U.S. Department of Agriculture
Economic Research Service
1800 M Street NW
Washington, DC 20036-5831
(202) 694-5050
E-mail: service@ers.usda.gov
URL: http://www.ers.usda.gov

U.S. Department of Agriculture
Food Safety and Inspection Service
FSIS Food Safety Education and Communications Staff
1400 Independence Ave. SW

Room 2932-South Bldg.
Washington, DC 20250-3700
(202) 720-7943
FAX: (202) 720-1843
E-mail: fsis.webmaster@usda.gov
URL: http://www.fsis.usda.gov

U.S. Department of Health and Human Services
Centers for Disease Control and Prevention
1600 Clifton Road
Atlanta, GA 30333
(800) 311-3435
URL: http://www.cdc.gov

U.S. Department of Health and Human Services
Food and Drug Administration
Center for Food Safety and Applied Nutrition
200 C St. SW
Washington, DC 20204
(202) 205-4850
(800) 332-4010
FAX: (202) 205-5025
URL: http://www.cfsan.fda.gov

Weight-control Information Network
1 Win Way
Bethesda, MD 20892-3665
(202) 828-1025
(202) 828-1028
FAX: (301) 984-7196
E-mail: win@info.niddk.nih.gov
URL: http://www.niddk.nih.gov/health/nutrit/nutrit.htm

Wheat Foods Council
10841 South Parker Rd., Suite 105
Parker, CO 80134
(303) 840- 8787
FAX: (303) 840-6877
E-mail: wfc@wheatfoods.org
URL: http://www.wheatfoods.org

RESOURCES

The U.S. Department of Agriculture (USDA) is responsible for collecting and reporting information on food in the United States. The Economic Research Service (ERS) of the USDA organizes much of that information, producing a wide range of valuable publications on agriculture and food. Their journal *FoodReview,* published three times a year, affords an excellent overview of domestic food consumption and expenditures, foreign aid, and food-assistance programs. *FoodReview's* Annual Spotlight on the U.S. Food System (1998) was an important resource in preparing this book. *Food Consumption, Prices, and Expenditures, 1970–1997* (1998) presents historical data on the per capita consumption of food and its cost. *Dietary Guidelines for Americans, 2000* was also an excellent resource.

The USDA National Agricultural Statistics Service conducted the *1997 Census of Agriculture* (1999), providing important data for this book. USDA's *Agricultural Baseline Projections to 2010* also provided useful information.

The USDA's *1996 Continuing Survey of Food Intakes by Individuals and Diet and Health Knowledge Survey* (1997), published by the Agricultural Research Service, is the government's main source of data on individual food intakes. The *Agriculture Fact Book 2000* (2000), produced by the Office of Communications, offers useful information about U.S. agriculture, rural America, nutrition, consumer issues, and trade.

The Bureau of Labor Statistics (BLS) of the Department of Labor examined how people spent their income in *Consumer Expenditures in 1999* (2000). The *Public Health Reports,* published bimonthly by the U.S. Department of Health and Human Services (HHS) and the Association of Schools of Public Health, discussed "The Selling of Olestra" (1998). The *Morbidity and Mortality Weekly Report,* prepared by the Centers for Disease Control and Prevention (CDC) of the HHS, periodically provides health studies and reports concerning nutrition.

The Food and Drug Administration (FDA) publishes agricultural information bulletins that provide useful articles on food safety and nutrition. The FDA's Pesticide Program *Residue Monitoring 1999* examined food safety. The Environmental Working Group has published data on children's exposure to pesticides in food.

PREVENTION(r) Magazine, with the Food Marketing Institute, produced *A Shopping for Health Report, 1998: A Look at the Self-Care Movement* (1998). In addition, the Food Marketing Institute published *Trends in the United States—Consumer Attitudes and the Supermarket, 2000,* a survey of supermarket shopping patterns. The Gale Group is grateful for their generous permission to reproduce their graphics.

Nutrition is an important issue for many Americans, and many newsletters address these concerns. The Center for Science in the Public Interest publishes *Nutrition Action Health Letter,* Tufts University puts out *The Tufts University Diet and Nutrition Letter,* and the University of California's School of Public Health publishes the *University of California at Berkeley Wellness Letter.* All of them provide useful information and current research on nutrition. Oklahoma State University graciously granted permission to use information on sources of fiber from its website.

The National Restaurant Association surveyed consumers in *Nutrition and Restaurants: A Consumer Perspective* (1993) and in *Meal Consumption Behavior* (1996). The Gale Group thanks the Association for permission to use its data. Gale Group is grateful to the Environmental Working Group for permission to reproduce graphics from *How 'Bout Them Apples?: Pesticides in Children's Food Ten Years After Alar* (1999). We also express our gratitude to the Wheat Foods Council for permission to reproduce graphics from their survey *Setting the Record Straight: What America Thinks About Fad Diets, Nutrition Advice and Food* (1999).

INDEX